VITAMINS

CW01496640

Rosemary Stanton is Australia's best-known nutritionist. She is the author of more than 20 books, appears frequently on television and radio, and contributes regular columns to many publications. In her consulting business she acts as an advisor to clients such as State and Commonwealth government departments, sports associations and teams, and selected sections of the food industry. She also lectures to medical students, doctors, nurses and teachers and is co-author (with Garry Egger) of the highly successful *Gutbuster* series.

VITAMINS

What they do and
what they *don't* do

Rosemary Stanton

ALLEN & UNWIN

First published in 1999 by
Allen & Unwin
9 Atchison Street
St Leonards NSW 1590
Australia
Phone: (61 2) 8425 0100
Fax: (61 2) 9906 2218
E-mail: frontdesk@allen-unwin.com.au
Web: http://www.allen-unwin.com.au

National Library of Australia
Cataloguing-in-Publication entry:

Stanton, Rosemary.
  Vitamins: what they do and what they don't do.

  Includes index.
  ISBN 1 86448 319 9.

  1. Vitamins in human nutrition. 2. Vitamins—Handbooks,
  manuals, etc. I. Title.

613.286

Set in 11/12.5 pt Garamond by DOCUPRO, Sydney
Printed and bound by Australian Print Group, Maryborough, Victoria

10 9 8 7 6 5 4 3 2 1

Contents

With thanks to Peter

Introduction

Vitamins are vitally important, as their name implies ('amine' means 'life'). There are thirteen of them: A, C, D, E, K, and eight members of the B complex. All are essential for health and energy, and to protect the body against many diseases.

Although vitamins are essential, it does not mean that more is necessarily better. Cars need petrol in their tanks but once the tank is full, adding more petrol will not improve performance. Instead, an excess of petrol will spill. It may do little more than contribute to waste, or it may damage paintwork and provide a fire hazard. Excess quantities of vitamins may also just be wasted, or may create havoc in the body. The fact that they are 'natural' does not make them safe. Nature produces many substances that are harmful and there is nothing we ingest that does not have a safe limit of intake.

The subject of vitamins can arouse strong feelings among those who line up their little bottles of pills to take each morning, and especially among those who market them. Some vitamin manufacturers sell their products in an ethical way, but some pill pushers assert that we can no longer rely on foods as sources of vitamins and state outright, or at least imply in their books and glossy brochures, that good health is impossible without their products. This is simply not true; analysis of ordinary fresh foods bought from stores and supermarkets confirms that more than sufficient quantities are easy to find, as long as you eat a variety of healthy foods.

If you try to live on a diet of confectionery, chips, cola drinks, alcohol, biscuits and junk foods, of course your diet will be deficient in vitamins. It will also lack many minerals, essential fatty acids, dietary fibre, protein and several thousand antioxidants. No amount of pill taking can make up for such a diet or counteract the harmful effects of a heap of saturated fat and junk ingredients. Such a diet needs basic changes and cannot be rescued with supplements.

Vitamins never come alone in food and their companion nutrients may be extremely important in the way the body uses any vitamin. This was not fully appreciated until studies discovered that supplements of beta carotene, normally found in foods with about 600 related substances, increased the incidence of lung cancer in smokers. In several other studies, beta carotene supplements were associated with an increase in bowel polyps, the first stage in bowel cancer. Yet many studies have shown that giving smokers fruits and vegetables (which contain beta carotene) helps protect against lung cancer, and the same foods are associated with a lower incidence of bowel polyps. Clearly, vitamins behave differently when they are isolated from their normal environment.

I am not against supplementary vitamins. They can be useful where people are unable or unwilling to eat normal foods. However, before using supplements, consumers need to know if their choice is appropriate, whether they are taking a lot or a little and what any side effects might be. This information is not always accessible and most vitamin supplements on sale in countries such as Australia do not tell you what percentage of the recommended daily intake of various vitamins they contain. At last examination, not a single multivitamin available in Australia contained the recommended daily intake of vitamins. Instead, products contained a lot of some vitamins and insignificant quantities of others. A cynic might point to the abundance of the cheaper vitamins and the scarcity of those that are more expensive. The composition, however, has little to do with the price the consumer pays. More expensive vitamins are not necessarily better. The subject of vitamin supplements is discussed more fully in Chapter 8.

In writing this book, I have tried to look at each of the vitamins, what they do in the body, where they are found, how to preserve them in cooking and food preparation, how much is desirable according to your age and stage of life, the effects of a deficiency, possible problems of an excess and current research findings.

The levels of recommended intakes of vitamins set by different countries sometimes vary slightly. This is because the figures are only ever averages based on estimates of human requirements. In Australia, the recommended dietary intakes (RDIs) have been set at levels designed to exceed the actual nutrient requirements of practically all healthy persons.

The values of nutrients listed for various foods are

given for typical servings. Those who eat more or less than these will need to take this into account if calculating their daily totals for any nutrient.

In this book each vitamin is discussed under headings. If you prefer to avoid the heavier material, skip the sections *What it is* and *Current research findings*. The detailed information in these sections is for those who want to delve more deeply into the subject.

Vitamins are measured in milligrams (mg) or micrograms (mcg or μg) and, occasionally, in the case of high-dose supplements, in grams. The unit used is set in each country to reduce the complexity of very large or small numbers. One gram equals 1000 milligrams and 1 milligram equals 1000 micrograms, so 1 gram equals 1 000 000 micrograms. The recommended dietary intake for vitamin A is listed as 750 micrograms. This could also be written as 0.75 milligrams or 0.00075 grams, but most people find it easier to cope with numbers without too many figures after a decimal point. For some vitamins, the term 'International Units' is also used. This usually compares the amount or the activity level of a vitamin with some standard. These terms are being phased out and have disappeared for some products. They still appear on some supplements and in some books.

1

Vitamin A and beta carotene

What it is

Vitamin A is not one substance but an umbrella term for a family of related compounds. Although we might think of a vitamin as a single compound, it often comprises a range of compounds. It is a bit like the way we talk in general about grass when the description 'grass' includes many different plants.

In 1914 Vitamin A was first found to be essential for the growth of rats, and its chemical structure was worked out in 1930. Research continues into all its functions and the way it acts within the body.

The parent vitamin A compound is called retinol, and most of our vitamin A comes either from preformed retinol (present in foods as a substance called retinyl ester) or is made in the body from some members of a family of plant pigments known as carotenoids, also discovered in 1930. In the body, synthesis from carotenoids mostly occurs in the wall of the intestine, although some can be made in the liver. There are more than 600 carotenoids which have various roles within the body, including their activity as antioxidants. Retinol itself does not function as an antioxidant.

About 50 of the members of the carotenoid family can be converted into vitamin A. The most widespread of these in foods is beta carotene. Every microgram of beta carotene can be converted to the equivalent of one-sixth of a microgram of vitamin A in the intestine. Although this does not sound like a high conversion rate, some foods contain so much beta carotene that they make a major contribution to total vitamin A. For example, a medium-sized carrot contains about 12 000 micrograms of beta carotene, which contributes 2000 micrograms of vitamin A, or almost three times the daily requirement.

For some of the other carotenoids, the efficiency of conversion to vitamin A is less than for beta carotene, and most are present in much smaller quantities in commonly consumed foods. Beta carotene and retinol, therefore, contribute most of the vitamin A in the diet. Retinol is the most efficient way to get vitamin A because it is better absorbed than beta carotene.

The other members of the carotenoid family were once considered unimportant but are now recognised by nutritionists as vitally important antioxidants. In fact, they are much more important in this role than beta carotene. The latest research shows that beta carotene is less effective as an antioxidant in humans than it is in other animals or in the test tube. Taking a supplement of beta carotene can therefore contribute to vitamin A, but is not particularly effective as a source of useful antioxidants. Eating foods that contain beta carotene is better than taking supplements as these foods also supply a good quantity of the hundreds of other antioxidant carotenoids. Beta carotene supplements do not contain the other carotenoids.

Vitamin A is a fat-soluble vitamin. This means that it needs fat for its absorption and can also be stored in body fat. It is not lost in the urine. A fat-soluble vitamin does not need to be taken every day because the body can store it. The disadvantage of this is that excess quantities can accumulate in body fat and may be toxic.

Preformed vitamin A, or retinol, is found only in animal foods. Fish liver oils and the liver of all animals are the richest sources. Polar bear liver is so high in vitamin A that some early explorers who ate the animal's liver died from vitamin A overdose. Other sources include egg yolk, fatty fish such as sardines and herring, butter, cheese, milk and other full-fat dairy products.

Low-fat dairy products do not contain vitamin A and this is the major reason why reduced-fat and skim milks must carry a warning label that they are not suitable for infants, except under medical supervision. Adults are more likely to ingest other sources of vitamin A, so these low-fat products are not a problem for them. Milk forms a major part of the diet for young children and few eat sufficient amounts of other foods that are rich in vitamin A.

Beta carotene comes mainly in brightly coloured fruits and vegetables, especially carrots (the similarity in the name reflects the strong connection). Although beta carotene is an orange colour, many green vegetables are also rich sources. In broccoli or spinach, for example, the colour of beta carotene is submerged beneath the green from the chlorophyll present. Beta carotene is also found in cod liver oil, red palm oil (used in parts of Asia) and egg yolk.

To be efficiently absorbed from the small intestine, both retinol and beta carotene require some dietary fat. Experts estimate that about 80 per cent of vitamin A is absorbed as long as the daily diet contains at least 10 grams of fat. This is not a problem for foods that provide retinol as they already contain fat. However, the vegetables that contain beta carotene have virtually no fat, so it is important to consume them with some form of fat; for example, with olive oil, as occurs in Mediterranean countries; stir-fried in sesame or other vegetable oil, as in many parts of Asia; with an oil-based salad dressing; or with meat, fish, chicken, nuts or eggs. Those who try to live on a no-fat diet, eating mainly fruits and vegetables, will not absorb much beta carotene.

What it does

Most children are told to eat their carrots so they will be able to see in the dark. This is not such a silly saying because vitamin A is intimately involved with vision. Retinol is taken up by cells in the eye, altered slightly and taken to the outer segment of the rods in the eye where it binds with a protein called opsin to form rhodopsin. When exposed to light, rhodopsin changes slightly and triggers a series of chemical reactions allowing good vision in dim light. Those who are deficient in vitamin A suffer from night blindness.

That vitamin A is essential can easily be seen from its roles within the body. It plays a part in the way cells divide in the body, especially during growth, and is involved in the first stages of cell differentiation in the development of an embryo after fertilisation has occurred. Vitamin A is also important in the formation of the surface layer of cells covering the skin and mucous surfaces within the body's organs and tissues, and the lining of blood vessels. It may also be important in the production of sperm, and plays a role in the body's immune response to infection and in the formation of bone. There is also evidence that vitamin A is essential for taste, hearing and appetite.

Beta carotene can function as an antioxidant, although the evidence is mounting that it may not serve this function to any extent in humans. The idea came from the many epidemiological studies showing that people who ate the most fruit and vegetables had the lowest incidence of many cancers and coronary heart disease. As fruits and vegetables are good sources of vitamins C, E and beta carotene, researchers initially thought these might be the reason for their protective effect.

After several trials, described later in this chapter and in chapters on the other relevant vitamins, beta carotene taken as a supplement proved not only to be ineffective, but to increase the incidence of some cancers. This does not apply to beta carotene obtained from fruits and vegetables.

How much you need

Because vitamin A comes from both retinol and beta carotene, the quantity in foods and the amount needed was once expressed as International Units (IU). One IU was determined by the biological activity of retinol or beta carotene in rats. The exact amount can now be measured so values in foods and in the body are expressed in micrograms. International Units are out-dated and can be ambiguous.

To take account of the contribution from retinol, beta carotene and other carotenoids, vitamin A is now expressed as retinol equivalents. One retinol equivalent = 1 microgram of retinol, or 6 micrograms of beta carotene, or 12 micrograms of other carotenoids.

If you are trying to compare the old IU values, 1 microgram of retinol = 3.3 IU of vitamin A activity from retinol, or 10 IU of vitamin A activity from beta carotene.

If you see the figures the other way round, 1 IU of retinol = 0.3 micrograms of retinol.

The Australian recommended dietary intake of vitamin A is as follows:

Age	RDI (micrograms retinol equivalents)
Breast-fed and bottle-fed	425
7–12 months	300
1–3 years	300
4–7 years	350
8–11 years	500
12–15 years	725
16–18 years	750
Adults, all ages	750
Pregnancy	750
Lactation	1200

Note: The RDI for adults has allowed a 50 per cent margin of safety over the mean estimated requirement.

The World Health Organisation (WHO) sets two recommended intakes for vitamin A. One is a basal level, defined as the amount needed to prevent any impairment of function that can be demonstrated clinically. For adult males, this is equivalent to 300 micrograms; for females 270 micrograms, with an additional 100 micrograms during pregnancy and 180 micrograms extra during lactation. WHO also sets a 'safe' level of 500 micrograms for females, 600 micrograms during pregnancy, 850 micrograms for lactating women and 600 micrograms for males over the age of twelve.

In the United Kingdom, three levels are described: a lower reference intake for those who have low needs; an estimated average requirement; and, a reference nutrient intake. These vary for adult men from 250 to 400 to 700 micrograms. For women, the corresponding values are 250, 400 and 600 micrograms. For pregnancy and lactation, levels are defined only in the higher category and these are 700 and 950 micrograms respectively.

In the United States, the recommended daily intake is 800 micrograms for women (1300 micrograms for the first six months of lactation, 1200 micrograms after that) and 1000 micrograms for men. These are higher than in other countries.

The different recommended intakes can be confusing, but the most significant factor is that recommended levels of intake of vitamin A in most categories are decreasing as research continues. The levels also vary according to estimates of average body weight. WHO figures are based on an average body weight of 55 kilograms for women and 65 kilograms for men. The UK estimates average weight for women of 60 kilograms and 74 kilograms for men while the USA works on the basis of 62 and 76 kilograms average weights for women and men.

Illness, especially if there is prolonged fever,

increases requirements. So does an inability to absorb fats from the diet, as may occur with certain serious and chronic liver conditions. The current vogue for liver cleansing diets does not mean that most people need more vitamin A. In fact, there is no physiological basis for using these diets and no evidence that most people have dirty livers that need cleansing.

Where it is found

As mentioned, vitamin A comes from preformed retinol in animal foods and from beta carotene in both animal and vegetable foods. The relative dominance of these sources of vitamin A varies from country to country. In Australia, much of the vitamin A comes from conversion of beta carotene, whereas in Scandinavian countries during winter when vegetables are expensive or scarce, retinol from products such as butter or cheese is more important.

In parts of Asia, most of the vitamin A comes from beta carotene, and if the diet is low in fat, as occurs in some areas, insufficient quantities are absorbed. Even though the diet theoretically has more than enough beta carotene, vitamin A deficiency still occurs.

Sources of retinol

The list of sources does not include most foods that have insignificant quantities, except where there is ignorance about the food. For example, unfortified soy beverage does not contain retinol or beta carotene and has been included to show that it is not equivalent to cow's milk in this respect. Fruits and vegetables not listed as sources of beta carotene generally do not contain significant quantities.

Food	Retinol (micrograms)
Dairy products	
Butter, 1 tablespoon, 20 g	175
Cheese, average of main varieties 50 g	160
Cheese, cottage, 50 g	40
Cheese, ricotta, 50 g	50
Cream, 50 g	195
Cream, clotted, 50 g	350
Fromage frais, fruit, 200 g	165
Fromage frais, low-fat, 200 g	5
Ice cream, vanilla, 2 small scoops	55
Malted-milk powder, 1 tablespoon	100
Milk, cow's, 1 cup, 250 mL	70
Milk, cow's, fat-reduced, 1 cup, 250 mL	35
Milk, cow's, skim, 1 cup, 250 mL	0
Milk, goat's, 1 cup, 250 mL	110
Milk, human, colostrum, 100 mL	155
Milk, human, mature, 100 mL	60
Milk, sheep's, 1 cup, 250 mL	205
Soy, beverage, 1 cup, 250 mL	0
Whey, 1 cup, 250 mL	10
Yoghurt, fruit, 200 g	50
Yoghurt, Greek, 200 g	230
Yoghurt, natural, 200 g	70
Yoghurt, sheep's milk, 200 g	170
Yoghurt, soy, 200 g	45
Fats	
Cod liver oil, 1 tablespoon, 20 g	360
Margarine, fortified, 20 g	170
Vegetable oils	0
Meat, poultry and eggs	
Black pudding, 50 g	425
Chicken, with skin, $\frac{1}{4}$	145
Chicken breast, no skin	trace

Food	Retinol (micrograms)
Devon sausage, 50 g	80
Egg, hen, 1	80
Egg, duck, 1	430
Liver, beef, cooked, 100 g	19 200
Liver, calves, cooked, 100 g	39 800
Liver, chicken, 100 g	12 200
Liver, lamb's fry, fried, 100 g	35 400
Beef, lamb, veal, pork	trace
Pâte de foie gras, 50 g	5400
Pâte, 50 g	3330
Sausage, cooked, 1 average, 140 g	25
Fish and seafood	
Anchovies, canned, 30 g	20
Crab, prawns, lobster	trace
Eel, 100 g	260–2500*
Fatty fish, such as gemfish, cooked, 200 g	440
Haddock, smoked, 150 g	90
Herring, grilled, 150 g	50
Kipper, cooked, 100 g	40
Mackerel, cooked, 150 g	70
Mullet, cooked, 150 g	90
Oysters, 12	90
Salmon, Atlantic, cooked, 200 g	35
Salmon, Pacific, cooked, 200 g	40–300
Salmon, pink, canned, 100 g	20
Salmon, red, canned, 100 g	50
Sardines, canned, 100 g	65
Squid, cooked, 100 g	15
Trout, rainbow, cooked, 200 g	60
Tuna, canned, 100 g	15
Tuna, fresh, cooked, 200 g	50
White fish, cooked, 200 g	15
Miscellaneous	
Chocolate, dark, 100 g	20

* Levels increase in older eels

Food	Retinol (micrograms)
Chocolate, milk, 100 g	95
Fish sauce, Hong Kong, 1 tablespoon	20
Liqueur, cream-based, 50 mL	85
Mayonnaise, 1 tablespoon	20
Ovaltine, 20 g	395
Oyster sauce, 1 tablespoon	20

Sources of beta carotene

Food	Beta carotene (micrograms)
Dairy products	
Butter, 1 tablespoon, 20 g	90
Cheese, average of main varieties 50 g	85
Cream, 50 g	130
Cream, clotted, 50 g	340
Ice cream, vanilla, 2 small scoops	55
Milk, 1 cup, 250 mL	50
Milk, goat's, 1 cup, 250 mL	trace
Milk, human, colostrum, 100 mL	135
Milk, human, mature, 100 mL	24
Soy, beverage, 1 cup, 250 mL	0
Whey, 1 cup, 250 mL	0
Yoghurt, fruit, 200 g	80
Yoghurt, natural, 200 g	40
Fats	
Margarine, fortified, 20 g	100
Red palm oil, unrefined, 1 tablespoon, 20 g	6000*
Meat and eggs	
Black pudding, 50 g	25
Egg, duck, 1	100
Kidney, lamb, cooked, 100 g	20

Food	Beta carotene (micrograms)
Liver, beef, cooked, 100 g	1920
Liver, calves, cooked, 100 g	100
Liver, chicken, 100 g	0
Liver, lamb's fry, fried, 100 g	60
Grain products	
Pasta, spinach, average serve, equal to 100 g dry	500
Pizza, $\frac{1}{2}$ medium, 300 g	500
Polenta, average serve, equal to 75 g dry	100
Fruit	
Apricots, 2 medium	565 (range 280–4700**)
Apricots, dried, 5 halves, 40 g, average	950
Babaco, 100 g	170
Banana, 1 medium	90
Blackberries, 150 g	120
Blackcurrants, raw, 100 g	100
Cape gooseberries, $\frac{1}{2}$ punnet, 100 g	1430
Cherries, raw, 150 g	110
Cumquat, 100 g	175
Feijoa, 1 medium	35
Figs, dried, 2	55
Fig, raw, 1 medium	150
Fruit salad, fresh, average, 1 cup	150
Gooseberries, 100 g	110
Grapefruit, $\frac{1}{2}$ medium	30
Grapefruit, pink, $\frac{1}{2}$ medium	310
Grapes, black, 150 g	105
Grapes, green sultana, 150 g	165
Guava, pink, 1 medium	515
Jackfruit, 150 g	1700
Kaki, 1 medium	1140
Kiwi fruit, 1 medium	70
Loquat, raw, 100 g	510
Mandarin, 1 medium	145
Mandarin oranges, canned, $\frac{1}{2}$ cup	120

Food	Beta carotene (micrograms)
Mango, 1 medium	3550
Mango, canned, $\frac{1}{2}$ cup	1500
Melon, honeydew, 200 g	80
Melon, rock, 200 g	1660
Nectarines, raw, 2 medium	165
Olives, black, 5, approx 25 g	10
Olives, green, 5, approx 25 g	45
Orange, blood, 1 medium	230
Orange, navel, 1 medium	140
Orange, valencia, 1 medium	200
Passionfruit, 2 medium	300
Pawpaw, ripe, 150 g	1365
Peach, canned, $\frac{1}{2}$ cup	85
Peach, white, 1 medium	80
Peach, yellow, 1 medium	150
Pepino, 1 medium	185
Persimmon, 1 medium	1000
Pineapple, 150 g	40
Pineapple, canned, $\frac{1}{2}$ cup	25
Plum, damson, 1	235
Plums, greengage, 2 medium	135
Plums, raw, 2 medium	225
Pomegranate, 1 medium	95
Prickly pear, 1 medium	45
Prunes, 6 medium	80–260
Quince, 1 medium	100
Rhubarb, stewed, 1 cup	75
Sapodilla, 1 medium	55
Tamarillo, 1 medium	840
Tangelo, 1 medium	420
Watermelon, 200 g	400
Juices and drinks	
Apricot nectar, 1 cup, 250 mL	825
Carrot juice, 250 mL	20 300

Food	Beta carotene (micrograms)
Orange and mango juice, 1 cup, 250 mL	245
Orange juice, purchased, 1 cup, 250 mL	250
Rose hip syrup, made up with water, 150 mL	150
Tomato juice, 1 cup, 250 mL	375
Vegetable juice, 1 cup, 250 mL	1225
Vegetables and vegetable-based products	
Amaranth leaves, raw, 50 g	840
Artichoke, globe, steamed, 1 medium	60
Asparagus, steamed, 6 spears	155
Asparagus, canned, 6 spears	120
Basil leaves, fresh, $\frac{1}{2}$ cup	1350
Beans, broad, cooked, 100 g	190
Beans, green, cooked, 1 cup	460
Beans, snake, cooked, average serve, 100 g	430
Broccoli, cooked, average serve, 100 g	475
Brussels sprouts, cooked, 6	195
Cabbage, Chinese, raw, 1 cup	150
Cabbage, green, cooked, 1 cup	100
Cabbage, mustard, raw, 1 cup	1300
Cabbage, red, raw, 1 cup	10
Capsicum, green, raw, $\frac{1}{2}$ medium	240
Capsicum, red, raw, $\frac{1}{2}$ medium	1840
Carrots, baby, 5	4380
Carrot, mature, 1 large	12 000
Cassava, boiled, 100 g	350
Cauliflower, cooked, 1 cup	60
Chicory, raw, 1 cup	180
Chilli, red hot, 1 small	800
Chinese greens, average, cooked, 1 cup	500
Chives, 1 tablespoon	175
Coriander leaves, $\frac{1}{2}$ cup	90
Cucumber, raw, $\frac{1}{2}$ cup	120
Curry leaves, fresh, 5	135
Eggplant, cooked, 100 g	70

Food	Beta carotene (micrograms)
Endive, raw, 1 cup	220
Kale, cooked, 1 cup	3375
Leek, sliced, cooked, 1 cup	720
Lettuce, cos, 3 leaves	430
Lettuce, iceberg, 3 leaves	80
Lettuce, mignonette, 3 leaves	520
Lettuce, average 3 outer dark green leaves	up to 2500
Okra, 3 small	500
Parsley, $\frac{1}{2}$ cup	1470
Parsley, Italian, $\frac{1}{2}$ cup	1185
Peas, green, 100 g	405
Peas, sugar snap (including pods), 100 g	695
Pumpkin, butternut, average serve, 120 g	3000
Pumpkin, nugget, average serve, 120 g	3650
Pumpkin, Queensland blue, average piece, baked, 150 g	4020
Rocket, 50 g	1000
Salad, mixed green, medium bowl	1500
Shallot, green, 3 medium	240
Silverbeet, average serving, 100 g	430
Spinach, English, raw, 100 g	3500
Spinach, frozen, 50 g portion	1920
Spring onion, 2 medium	440
Squash, scallopini, 2 medium	600
Sweet corn, 1 cob	360
Sweet corn kernels, canned or frozen, $\frac{1}{2}$ cup	70
Sweet potato, orange, medium piece, baked, 150 g	6000***
Taro leaves, 50 g	3500
Tomato, 1 medium, 150 g	500–1000**
Tomatoes, cherry, $\frac{1}{2}$ punnet	610
Tomatoes, egg, 2 medium, 150 g	430
Tomato paste, 1 tablespoon	265
Tomato puree, $\frac{1}{2}$ cup	550–800
Tomatoes, sun-dried, 20 g	80

Food	Beta carotene (micrograms)
Vine leaves, preserved, 6	500
Watercress, 50 g	1000
Zucchini, golden, 2 small	130
Zucchini, green, 2 small	400
Legumes	
Baked beans, canned, 1 cup	140
Chickpeas, cooked, 1 cup	45
Dried herbs and spices	
Basil, 1 teaspoon	280
Chilli powder, 1 teaspoon	1050
Coriander, 1 teaspoon	400
Curry powder, 1 teaspoon	720
Dill, 1 teaspoon	1660
Marjoram, 1 teaspoon	240
Mint, 1 teaspoon	240
Oregano, 1 teaspoon	200
Paprika, 1 teaspoon	1810
Parsley, 1 teaspoon	1080
Rosemary, 1 teaspoon	95
Tarragon, 1 teaspoon	125
Thyme, 1 teaspoon	115
Nuts and seeds	
Pepitas (roasted pumpkin seeds), 50 g	115
Pistachio nuts, 50 g	65
Miscellaneous	
Chilli sauce, 1 tablespoon	115
Chocolate, milk, 100 g	20
Liqueur, cream-based, 50 mL	45
Mayonnaise, 1 tablespoon	20
Pasta sauce, tomato, commercial, $\frac{3}{4}$ cup	490
Pasta sauce, tomato, homemade, $\frac{3}{4}$ cup	600
Seaweed, nori, average serve, 10 g	1500
Tabbouli, 1 cup	1200

Food	Beta carotene (micrograms)
Tempeh, 100 g	30
Tomato sauce, 1 tablespoon	50
Tomato soup, canned with added milk, 1 cup	500

* Also contains 4800 micrograms alpha carotene which equates to 400 micrograms retinol

** Depending on variety. Deeper coloured fruit has higher levels

*** Beta carotene can be as high as 16 000 micrograms per 100 grams in deep orange sweet potato

Note: Each microgram of beta carotene is equivalent to one-sixth of a microgram of vitamin A.

Other carotenoids

In most foods, the levels of alpha carotene, alpha and beta cryptoxanthin, zeaxanthin, lutein and lycopene are too small to make much of a contribution to vitamin A, although the quantities present are more than adequate to act as efficient antioxidants. Because they do not contribute significantly to vitamin A levels, these other carotenoids have not been measured in the past. However, with their importance as antioxidants now being recognised, this is being rectified.

Both carrots and pumpkin contain significant quantities of alpha carotene, which make an important contribution to the retinol equivalents of these foods (around 2000 micrograms which equates to about 165 micrograms retinol). Red capsicum and passionfruit also contribute smaller, but still significant quantities.

Sources of beta cryptoxanthin are not generally great enough to make a large contribution to vitamin A but are useful for antioxidant capacity.

Sources of beta cryptoxanthin

Food	Beta cryptoxanthin (micrograms)
Fruit	
Cumquat, 1	45
Guava, 1 average	110
Loquats, 4 average size	100
Mango, 1 medium	50
Passionfruit, pulp, 2 tablespoons	150
Pawpaw, 150 g slice	2050
Persimmon, 1 medium	1500
Tamarillo, 1 medium	675
Vegetables	
Amaranth leaves, 1 cup	45
Capsicum, red, $\frac{1}{2}$	1500
Carrots, baby, raw, 100 g	190
Carrots, cooked, 100 g	55
Spinach, average serve	40
Sweet corn, cob	160
Sweet corn, kernels, $\frac{1}{2}$ cup	180
Tomato, 1 average	50

Herbs
Fenugreek seeds, stone fruits and citrus also provide some.
Zeaxanthin is found principally in spinach. It has a specific beneficial action on the eye and high intakes have been associated with reduced incidence of cataracts.

Sources of lycopene

The major sources of lycopene, another important anti-oxidant, are tomatoes, which contain 1075 micrograms per 100 grams. Lycopene is absorbed better from cooked tomato products such as tomato puree, canned tomatoes, tomato sauce and pasta sauces featuring tomatoes.

Watermelon, pink grapefruit, apricot and red palm oil are also sources of lycopene.

Effect of cooking

Cooking does not significantly decrease levels of retinol in food. Some beta carotene can be leached out of foods cooked in water for extended periods (when boiling carrots the water becomes orange), but cooking losses are not great. Cooking losses are greater for some carotenoids, such as alpha carotene, whereas others, such as lycopene, are made more available to the body by cooking. As always, variety is important and eating some raw and some cooked foods makes good sense. In general though, cooking has minimal effects on vitamin A.

Deficiency

In many parts of the world, vitamin A deficiency is a major problem with up to 100 million children suffering from it. In addition, researchers estimate that 500 000 preschool children go blind each year from a lack of this essential vitamin. The first sign of their vitamin A deficiency is foamy white spots (called Bitot's spots) in the conjunctiva of the eye. Among adults, vitamin A deficiency generally occurs in lactating women.

Vitamin A deficiency is usually linked with insufficient food after weaning, especially foods that provide protein and fat. As discussed earlier, some fat is required for absorption of both retinol and beta carotene. In parts of the world where there may be an ample supply of vegetables containing beta carotene but few available sources of dietary fat, the beta carotene is not absorbed. Vitamin A deficiency is rare in countries such as Australia where children and adults have access to dairy products which provide vitamin A as retinol and beta carotene as well as fat to assist in their absorption. However, it is occasionally seen in severe liver disease, especially in chronic alcoholics and usually in association with zinc deficiency. (Zinc deficiency also causes night blindness because the enzyme that enables retinol to be converted to the form needed by the eye also requires zinc.)

There is no single simple way to measure vitamin A levels in the body as it is present in so many tissues. However, researchers now have confidence in a technique that uses total isotope dilution methods to measure total body reserves of vitamin A.

People with insulin-dependent diabetes have lower levels of vitamin A in their blood serum. This is not due to any dietary deficiency and there is no impairment of retinol absorption with diabetes. Researchers think the problem is a difficulty in transporting vitamin A from its storage areas in the liver to other areas of the body, such as the retina in the eye. Treatment with insulin seems to help the problem but giving vitamin A supplements could make it worse because liver stores of the vitamin could increase to toxic levels. The lower levels of vitamin A are not the reason for eye problems in people with diabetes; these are due to damage to the small blood vessels in the retina from high levels of glucose in the blood.

Excess

Vitamin A is stored in the liver and the body usually has enough for more than a year's supply. Large quantities of retinol are toxic. Large amounts of beta carotene are not considered toxic if they come from food, although they will cause a yellowing of the skin, especially on the palms of the hand. High-dose supplements of beta carotene are not toxic but several trials have now found increased incidence of lung cancer and bowel polyps (the first stage of bowel cancer) in those taking beta carotene supplements. The difference in toxicity almost certainly comes from the fact that beta carotene only occurs in nature with large numbers of other carotenoids, many of which provide protection against various cancers. In supplements it comes alone and there is a suggestion that, under such circumstances, it may interfere with the absorption of the other protective carotenoids in foods. There is also the chance that large doses of beta carotene may act as a growth factor for cancerous cells that may be silently present in the body.

A single large dose of retinol of 100 times the RDI for adults, or 20 times the RDI for infants, can produce acute toxicity with symptoms that include nausea, vomiting, dizziness, headaches, blurred vision and an inability to coordinate muscular movements. In extreme cases, these symptoms can progress to drowsiness, drying and flaking skin, haemorrhage, convulsions, coma and death. Such cases are rare and most cases of inadvertent poisoning with a single large dose recover within a couple of weeks.

A chronic oversupply of vitamin A is much more common and can occur in those who take supplementary vitamin A of even ten times the RDI. Symptoms include headache, hair loss, pains in the joints and bones, dry and itchy skin and, clinically, an enlarged liver. Just as some people may need more than minimal quantities of vitamin A, so others seem to be unable to tolerate even a moderate chronic overdose. This appears to be genetic and symptoms have been reported in those taking as little as 1800 to 16 000 micrograms a day.

It is vitally important for women of child-bearing age to avoid excess vitamin A because a chronic dose of even a small amount surplus to the body's requirements increases the chances of birth defects. These can include early spontaneous abortion, gross abnormalities in the foetus and permanent learning disability in those that survive birth. Drugs related to vitamin A and used for treating acne have been responsible for most cases, but all multivitamin supplements that contain vitamin A must now carry a warning label about the risks during pregnancy. Many brands have simply dropped the vitamin A from their supplements altogether. Health authorities also recommend that pregnant women limit their daily intake of retinol from all sources (food and supplements) to 2400 micrograms. There is no evidence that large quantities of beta carotene are toxic during pregnancy.

Beta carotene supplements

We have always assumed that beta carotene was harmless and this assumption still holds for beta carotene in foods. However, there are now at least five trials where supplements of beta carotene that were expected to confer benefits, had the opposite effect. These trials were all well designed and well controlled and several had to be stopped early because of the ethics of continuing with a trial where people taking beta carotene supplements had worse health outcomes and higher death rates than those taking placebo pills. Beta carotene was used in these trials because epidemiological studies showed that those who ate the most fruit and vegetables had the lowest risk of death from problems such as coronary heart disease, stroke, lung and bowel cancers. Researchers assumed it was the vitamins in these foods that were protective.

In one major trial of 29 000 Finnish male smokers, deaths from coronary heart disease and stroke, as well as deaths from lung cancer, were significantly greater in those given supplements of beta carotene. Critics claim that these results were to be expected, given that the men were smokers, but numerous studies show that smokers who eat more fruits and vegetables have significantly less lung cancer and heart disease. A follow-up study on survivors in this trial has shown an increase in angina in those who had taken beta carotene.

Over 22 000 men in the Physician's Health Study in the United States who took beta carotene supplements every second day for 12 years had no reduction in heart disease, cancers, fatal heart attacks or total mortality. While this gives some comfort that they were not doing any harm, it is a clear indication that taking extra beta carotene does not do any good.

In the CARET trial (Beta Carotene And Retinol Efficacy Trial), 18 000 smokers, former smokers and asbestos workers taking 30 milligrams beta carotene and 25 000 IU retinol palmitate had a 28 per cent higher risk of lung cancer and 46 per cent more deaths from lung cancer than those not taking the supplements. They also had 17 per cent higher total mortality and 26 per cent higher death rate from cardiovascular disease. The ethics committee demanded that the trial be stopped because of the gravity of its results.

Two major trials, including one in Australia, gave

beta carotene supplements to those who had already had a bowel polyp, and were therefore at high risk of another and of subsequent bowel cancer. Once again, the supplements gave the wrong results and this aspect of the trials had to be stopped.

Studies giving beta carotene to try to prevent pre-malignant lesions likely to lead to oral cancers also failed.

With results like these it is unlikely that any ethics committees will give permission for more trials of beta carotene supplements, and we must conclude that such supplements are potentially hazardous. Some researchers now suggest that beta carotene supplements should carry a notice warning that they could be harmful. Others mourn the wastage of millions of dollars of research money.

Beta carotene is a good example of how a great deal of favourable publicity is worse than useless if clinical trials to prove the hype have not been done. Greenberg and Sporn, two prominent researchers into the effects of antioxidant vitamins, have stated that we 'should put to rest any remaining hopes that, for adults, beta carotene supplements may be an effective means of lowering the risk of cancer and cardiovascular disease'.

There is no suggestion that foods rich in beta carotene cause any problems. Dozens of studies show that those who eat more of these foods—fruits and vegetables—are well protected against many cancers. It is unlikely that the protection comes from the food's content of beta carotene.

Current research findings

Apart from issues already discussed, much of the research in the area of vitamin A concerns carotenoids that are not significant for their ability to be converted to vitamin A, but have an important role in preventing chronic diseases such as various cancers and cataracts. Not all of the 600 or so carotenoids are currently being investigated, but many are, especially lycopene, zeaxanthin and alpha carotene. Beta carotene has been extensively researched as an antioxidant, and this research is continuing. However, the use of resources for such research is strange in light of the continued failure of beta carotene as an effective antioxidant in humans.

There is also some doubt about the efficiency with which beta carotene from some sources is converted to vitamin A in the body. It is likely that the calculations used to translate the intake of beta carotene to retinol equivalents may change for some foods where the absorption and conversion is less efficient.

2

Vitamin B

The B complex consists of eight different vitamins, with numbers ranging from B_1 to B_{12}. There are gaps in the numbering system and some members of the complex have never been assigned a number. The gaps have occurred because compounds once thought to be part of the vitamin B complex were later found not to be vitamins and so were removed. Each vitamin in the complex now has a distinct name, although, in common usage, some of the subscripts have stuck.

All the B complex vitamins, with the exception of B_{12}, are soluble in water. Apart from B_{12} and folate, both of which can be stored to some extent in the liver, any excess quantities of the B vitamins are lost in the urine. Contrary to popular belief, this does not mean that large doses of some members of the complex don't have undesirable or toxic effects in the body. Before excess quantities are excreted, some can do damage. Some can also interfere with each other, especially folate and vitamin B_{12}. The old idea that the quantities of water-soluble B complex vitamins are irrelevant is therefore not correct.

THIAMIN OR VITAMIN B₁

What it is

This was the vitamin that started vitamins. A disease known from ancient Chinese literature to date from 2600 BC was first fully described by a Dutch doctor working in Java in 1630. He called the disease beriberi, which means 'sheep', because sufferers were said to walk like sheep. By 1882, a Japanese naval officer decided the staggering gait, loss of reflexes, lack of muscle coordination and memory defects must have something to do with diet since the symptoms were common in sailors whose rations consisted of little more than polished rice. When given meat, bread and vegetables, sailors did not experience these symptoms.

It was another Dutch doctor, working in Java in 1897, who described beriberi in chickens and recognised that something present in unpolished rice could prevent it. Chickens fed polished rice became diseased whereas those consuming unpolished rice stayed healthy.

In 1911, a scientist with the unlikely name of Dr Funk, working on the magic factor in rice polishings coined the term 'vitamine'. 'Vita' means 'life', and Dr Funk and others of the time thought the molecule also held one of the nitrogen-containing substances called 'amines' (hence vit*amine* and thi*amine*). By 1936, the structure of thiamin and its role were elucidated and scientists found that amines were not involved in its structure. They therefore dropped the 'e' from the word.

However, many people retained the 'amine' portion of thiamine, and some computer spell-check programs and the labels on some foods and supplements still add the 'e'. The correct spelling is thiamin. It is also known as aneurin.

What it does

Like many members of the B complex, thiamin takes part in the complex processes whereby the body extracts energy from carbohydrates and fats, and also from products formed during the metabolism of branched chain amino acids (components of protein). More recently, thiamin has been identified as vital in conducting impulses within nervous tissue. In fish with electric organs, thiamin helps in their amazing functioning.

As part of the chain of reactions contributing energy to the body, thiamin plays a role in producing sugars called pentoses. When thiamin levels in the body are low, this activity decreases in red blood cells and can be measured as an indication of a deficiency of the vitamin. Modern methods including high-performance liquid chromatography can be used to measure levels of thiamin in foods and in the blood. Low urinary levels of thiamin collected over a 24-hour period after taking a large dose also indicate a deficiency.

How much you need

The more carbohydrate and alcohol you consume, the more thiamin you need. Daily requirements are usually linked to energy intake, with 0.08 milligrams of thiamin needed for every 1000 kilojoules of energy intake. To take account of individual variation in needs, the National Health and Medical Research Council has increased the recommended level to 0.1 milligrams per 1000 kilojoules. For pregnancy, an extra amount has been included for the baby's needs as well as for the mother's increased energy intake.

The body does not store much thiamin, so it is needed regularly. Large doses taken as an occasional supplement are not well absorbed.

The recommended dietary intake of thiamin is as follows:

Age	RDI (milligrams)
Breast-fed	0.15
Bottle-fed	0.25
7–12 months	0.35
1–3 years	0.5
4–7 years	0.7
Boys, 8–11 years	0.9
Girls, 8–11 years	0.8
Boys, 12–15 years	1.2
Girls, 12–15 years	1.0
Boys, 16–18 years	1.2
Girls, 16–18 years	0.9
Men, 19–64 years	1.1
Men, over 64 years	0.9
Women, 19–54 years	0.8
Women, over 54 years	0.7
Pregnancy	1.0
Lactation	1.2

Where it is found

The best sources of thiamin are Vegemite, pork, some nuts, wholegrain and enriched cereals, salmon, breads, legumes and seeds. Fruits and vegetables contain only small quantities.

Food	Thiamin (milligrams)
Breads, grains and cereals	
Barley, pearl, cooked, 1 cup, 180 g	0.40
Bran, oat, 1 tablespoon, 15 g	0.18
Bran, rice, 1 tablespoon, 15 g	0.45
Bran, wheat, 1 tablespoon, 8 g	0.06
Bread, multigrain, 1 slice, 30 g	0.12
Bread, white, enriched, 1 slice, 30 g	0.10–0.33
Bread, wholemeal, 1 slice, 30 g	0.12
Burghul (cracked wheat), soaked, $\frac{1}{2}$ cup, 100g	0.46
Flour, white, 1 cup, 125 g	0.34
Flour, wholemeal, 1 cup, 130 g	0.53
Millet flour, 1 cup, 130 g	0.88
Muffin, English, toasted, 1, 60 g	0.19
Oats, rolled, raw, $\frac{1}{2}$ cup, 50 g	0.27
Pasta, cooked, 1 cup, 180 g	0.04
Pasta, egg noodles, cooked, 1 cup, 180 g	0.09
Pasta, wholemeal, cooked, 1 cup, 180 g	0.38
Polenta, cooked, 1 cup, 200 g	0.41
Rice, brown, cooked, 1 cup, 180 g	0.25
Rice, sungold, cooked, 1 cup, 180 g	0.11
Rice, white, cooked, 1 cup, 180 g	0.15
Rye flour, 1 cup, 130 g	0.52
Wheat germ, 1 tablespoon, 10 g	0.14
Breakfast cereals	
Allbran, $\frac{1}{2}$ cup, 40 g	0.38
Branflakes, average serve, 45 g	0.59
Cornflakes, average serve, 40 g	0.72
Muesli, natural, average serve, 60 g	0.58
Muesli, toasted, average serve, 60 g	0.55
Oats, rolled, cooked, average serve, 300 g	0.24
Semolina, cooked, 1 cup, 180 g	0
Weetbix, 2 biscuits, 30 g	0.55
Dairy products	
Cheese, average of main varieties, 50 g	0.01

Food	Thiamin (milligrams)
Milk, cow's, 1 cup	0.13
Milk, goat's, 1 cup	0.10
Milk, sheep's, 1 cup	0.20
Milk, skim, 1 cup	0.10
Soy, beverage, fortified, 250 mL	0.15
Soy, beverage, unfortified, 250 mL	0.53
Yoghurt, natural or fruit, 200 g	0.20
Meat, poultry and eggs	
Bacon, grilled, 2 rashers, 60 g	0.40
Beef or veal, cooked, average serve, 150 g	0.15
Chicken, cooked, $\frac{1}{4}$ medium	0.11
Egg, hen, boiled, 1	0.04
Fish, average fillet, grilled, 200 g	0.22
Kidney, lamb, 100 g	0.45
Lamb, cooked, average serve, 150 g	0.11
Liver, cooked, 100 g	0.20
Pork, cooked, average serve, 150 g	0.96
Fish and seafood	
Prawns, cooked, 6 medium	0.02
Salmon, grilled, 200 g	0.50
Salmon, pink or red, canned, 100 g	0.02
Sardines, canned, 100 g	0.01
Nuts and seeds	
Almonds, 50 g	0.07
Brazil nuts, 50 g	0.30
Cashews, 50 g	0.29
Chestnuts, 50 g	0.07
Coconut, fresh, 50 g	0.02
Hazelnuts, 50 g	0.20
Macadamias, 50 g	0.14
Peanut butter, 1 tablespoon	0.03
Peanuts, raw with skin, 50 g	0.40
Peanuts, roasted and salted, 50 g	0.18

Food	Thiamin (milligrams)
Pecans, 50 g	0.21
Pine nuts, 50 g	0.29
Pistachios, 50 g	0.29
Pumpkin seeds, 1 tablespoon	0.05
Sesame seeds, 2 teaspoons	0.10
Sunflower seeds, 1 tablespoon	0.32
Tahini paste, 1 tablespoon	0.19
Walnuts, 50 g	0.17
Fruit	
Average piece, fresh	0.06
Sultanas or raisins, 50 g	0.08
Vegetables	
Asparagus, steamed, 6 spears	0.10
Beans, broad, cooked, 100 g	0.17
Broccoli, cooked, average serve, 100 g	0.07
Brussels sprouts, cooked, 6	0.08
Cabbage, green, cooked, 1 cup	0.06
Cabbage, mustard, raw, 1 cup	0.06
Cabbage, red, cooked, 1 cup	0.12
Capsicum, green, raw, $\frac{1}{2}$ medium	0.02
Capsicum, red, raw, $\frac{1}{2}$ medium	0.03
Carrot, mature, cooked, 1 medium	0.11
Carrot, mature, raw, 1 medium	0.12
Cassava, boiled, 100 g	0.13
Cauliflower, cooked, 1 cup	0.08
Celeriac, cooked, 100 g	0.13
Celery, raw, 100 g	0.06
Leeks, cooked, 1 average	0.03
Lettuce, 2 leaves	0.08
Mushrooms, canned, 100 g	0.02
Mushrooms, raw, 100 g	0.09
Onion, cooked, 100 g	0.09
Onion, raw, 100 g	0.13
Parsley, $\frac{1}{2}$ cup	0.02

Food	Thiamin (milligrams)
Peas, green, cooked, 100 g	0.23
Pumpkin, butternut, average serve, 120 g	0.08
Pumpkin, nugget, average serve, 120 g	0.05
Snow peas, cooked, 100 g	0.14
Spinach, Chinese, raw, 100 g	0.20
Spinach, English, cooked, 100 g	0.05
Sweet corn, cooked, 1 cob	0.15
Tomato, 1 medium, 150 g	0.06
Tomato, egg, 2 medium, 150 g	0.09
Zucchini, 1 average	0.10
Legumes	
Baked beans, canned, 1 cup	0.10
Beans, haricot, cooked, 1 cup	0.16
Beans, kidney, cooked, 1 cup	0.20
Soy beans, cooked, 1 cup	0.20
Split peas, cooked, 1 cup	0.22
Take-away foods	
Barbecued chicken, $\frac{1}{4}$	0.08
Big breakfast, 1 serve	0.02
Chiko roll, 1	0.13
Chips, average serve, 150 g	0.11
Corn chips, 50 g	0.06
Fish, battered and fried, 1 piece, 150 g	0.14
Garlic bread, 2 slices	0.04
Hamburger, 1	0.10
Hamburger, fast food chain, 1	0.53
Meat pie, 1	0.09
Pizza, $\frac{1}{2}$ medium, average, 300 g	0.20
Potato crisps, 50 g	0.06
Sausage roll, 1	0.08
Thickshake, chocolate, 300 mL	0.15
Juices	
Orange juice, 250 mL	0.13

Food	Thiamin (milligrams)
Miscellaneous	
Bonox, 1 teaspoon	0.01
Chocolate, 50 g	0.06
Malted-milk powder, 1 tablespoon	0.44
Marmite, 1 teaspoon	0.55
Muesli bar, 1, 60 g	0.07
Ovaltine, 2 teaspoons	0.31
Vegemite, 1 teaspoon	0.90

Effect of cooking

Heat and water used during cooking destroy thiamin and the combination of moist heat is particularly destructive. For example, when bread is toasted, about 20 per cent of the thiamin is lost, but when vegetables and products such as pasta are boiled in water, or semolina is cooked into a porridge, losses may be much greater. Some of the thiamin will be present in the water used to cook vegetables, and using this in soups or sauces helps reduce losses.

Some foods also contain enzymes, called thiaminases, that destroy thiamin. Thiaminases are found in the intestine of carp and some other fish, and also in ferns considered delicacies in parts of Japan. Commonly consumed foods such as blueberries, black-currants, red cabbage, brussels sprouts, beetroot and tea also contain polyphenols that are valuable in many ways, but may inactivate some of the thiamin from foods consumed at the same time. In practice, thiaminases are partially destroyed by cooking and would only be a problem if one or more of these foods made up the major part of the diet. However, if chickens or cats are given fish meal or foods made from carp as their major diet, they can develop a paralysis of the legs due to thiamin deficiency.

Deficiency

There are several ways that thiamin deficiency can develop. In less-developed parts of the world, the most common is a simple deficiency that occurs with a diet consisting mainly of highly refined cereal or grain products. Adding sugar, sugary foods or fat makes a dietary deficiency worse, as these foods do not contribute any thiamin and increase the amount required. Those with anorexia nervosa who eat very little and confine their meagre portions to sweets or foods high in refined sugars have a higher than normal risk of thiamin deficiency.

The major cause of thiamin deficiency in developed countries is a diet high in alcohol. In an effort to combat this, thiamin is now added by law to some staple grain-based products to replace the losses caused by processing. In many countries, including Australia, the food selected has been flour used for making bread. Preliminary data show that the addition of thiamin seems to be decreasing the incidence of thiamin deficiency.

Another way to develop thiamin deficiency is from a restricted diet containing foods high in thiaminases. This is not common.

In all types of thiamin deficiency, the first symptoms are tiredness and headache. However, these symptoms may have many other causes and are not specific to a lack of thiamin. Before frank beriberi occurs, changes in the heart and nervous system are apparent. The heart rate increases, breathing is difficult and fluid may accumulate in the legs. Tendon reflexes are exaggerated, muscles become weak, the feet feel like they are burning and convulsions may occur. Eventually, thiamin deficiency leads to Wernicke's encephalopathy and Korsakoff's psychosis, conditions named after the scientists who first described these serious problems seen in chronic alcoholics. Abnormalities that develop in the brain lead to confusion, amnesia and coma. By giving alcoholics thiamin, either added to foods or as a supplement, these symptoms can be avoided. Once signs of serious deficiency are present, thiamin is usually given by injection.

Foetal alcohol syndrome, characterised by retarded growth of the baby within the uterus, congenital malformations and abnormalities in development after birth, occurs in babies of women who drink heavily during pregnancy. The syndrome is due to lack of thiamin.

Excess

Thiamin is one of the safest vitamins if given orally. However, very large oral doses may cause gastric upset and injections of thiamin of 100–200 times the recommended dietary intake and given intramuscularly have been reported to cause shock. In general, with the doses available, thiamin is safe. Excess intake is a waste of money rather than a hazard.

Thiamin supplements

In chronic alcoholism, thiamin supplements in large doses are essential for recovery. However, this cannot be extrapolated to assume that anyone who has a drink or two should take extra thiamin. It has no effect on a hangover. Most people eating a normal varied diet in developed countries will not benefit from extra thiamin and the fact that some multivitamins contain many times the recommended intake is probably because it is cheap and relatively harmless. There is no evidence that taking extra thiamin above the body's needs has any benefits, except for chronic alcoholics, and the profitability of those selling vitamins.

Current research findings

Most research into thiamin is concerned with the effects of a deficiency in chronic alcoholism and working out ways to fortify suitable foods with thiamin. This is especially important in parts of the world where people have little food. The vitamin is cheap and can easily be added to foods without changing their essential character.

RIBOFLAVIN OR VITAMIN B₂

What it is

If you take a multivitamin and then burp afterwards, the taste in your mouth comes from riboflavin. It is also responsible for the intensely greenish-yellow coloured urine you pass soon after taking a multivitamin. Riboflavin is highly fluorescent yellow and only a small amount (a maximum of 25 milligrams) can be absorbed. Anything over that quantity is excreted in urine.

Riboflavin is less soluble in water than most of its relatives in the B complex. It is also highly sensitive to light. That is why milk, a major source of riboflavin, should not be stored in clear containers under fluorescent lights. High levels of acidity, alkalinity or light can also break down riboflavin to a form that is biologically inactive.

For those who want to know the chemistry, the riboflavin molecule belongs in the isoalloxane family and is 7,8-dimethyl–10-(1'-D-ribityl) isoalloxane. If you prefer absolute simplicity, riboflavin is called vitamin B_2 and it exists in many forms in foods.

What it does

Like other vitamins of the B complex, riboflavin is involved in the release of energy from food. It is also a powerful antioxidant. Once riboflavin is absorbed from the upper part of the small intestine, it combines with particular proteins to form flavin mononucleotide and flavin adenine dinucleotide. These active forms of riboflavin are needed by enzymes that release energy from foods. Riboflavin is essential for growth and also to keep the nervous system, eyes and skin healthy.

Absorption of the vitamin is increased by the presence of food in the intestine. Food slows down the emptying of the stomach and this gives a longer time for the riboflavin to be absorbed. This can be important in those who need supplements, which should always be taken with a meal. Psyllium gum, used in some breakfast cereals and fibre supplements, decreases the rate of riboflavin absorption. Wheat bran and other types of dietary fibre do not seem to have the same effect.

Alcohol impairs absorption of riboflavin and also its conversion into its active forms. Thus, riboflavin deficiency is common in chronic alcoholics.

Copper, zinc, iron, caffeine, theophylline (found in tea and coffee), saccharine, tryptophan (an amino acid found in protein-rich foods) and vitamins C and nicotinamide (a form of vitamin B_3) can all form complexes with riboflavin and affect its bioavailability. Whether this is important in the context of an adequate dietary intake is not known.

How much you need

Recommended intakes are related to energy requirements, with quantities being set as 0.1 milligrams of riboflavin for every 1000 kilojoules, plus an extra 50 per cent safety margin. Larger quantities are excreted in the urine.

There is some evidence that physical activity increases riboflavin needs, although most athletes get plenty from their diet. Less riboflavin is needed by the body during sleep so those who sleep for only a few hours a night may have higher requirements. However, to complicate this, those confined to bed for prolonged periods tend to excrete more riboflavin.

The recommended dietary intake of riboflavin is as follows:

Age	RDI (milligrams)
Breast-fed and bottle-fed	0.4
7–12 months	0.6
1–3 years	0.8
4–7 years	1.1
Boys, 8–11 years	1.4
Girls, 8–11 years	1.3
Boys, 12–15 years	1.8
Girls, 12–15 years	1.6
Boys, 16–18 years	1.9
Girls, 16–18 years	1.4
Men, 19–64 years	1.7
Men, over 64 years	1.3

Age	RDI (milligrams)
Women, 19–54 years	1.2
Women, over 54 years	1.0
Pregnancy	1.5
Lactation	1.7

Where it is found

The richest sources of riboflavin are liver, kidney, Vegemite and Marmite. Dairy products (milk, cheeses and yoghurt), breakfast cereals with added riboflavin, meats, some seafood and some nuts are also major sources. Fruits contain only small quantities. Mushrooms are a good source.

Food	Riboflavin (milligrams)
Breads, grains and cereals	
Bran, oat, 1 tablespoon, 15 g	0.03
Bran, rice, 1 tablespoon, 15 g	0.08
Bran, wheat, 1 tablespoon, 8 g	0.02
Bread, multigrain, 1 slice, 30 g	0.03
Bread, white, 1 slice, 30 g	0.02
Bread, wholemeal, 1 slice, 30 g	0.04
Flour, white, 1 cup, 125 g	0.19
Flour, wholemeal, 1 cup, 130 g	0.14
Millet flour, 1 cup, 130 g	0.25
Muffin, English, toasted, 1, 60 g	0.08
Oats, rolled, raw, $\frac{1}{2}$ cup, 50 g	0.05
Pasta, egg noodles, cooked, 1 cup, 180 g	0.04
Pasta, wholemeal, cooked, 1 cup, 180 g	0.13
Rice, brown, cooked, 1 cup, 180 g	0.04
Rye flour, 1 cup, 130 g	0.08
Wheat germ, 1 tablespoon, 10 g	0.06
Breakfast cereals	
Allbran, $\frac{1}{2}$ cup, 40 g	0.48

Food	Riboflavin (milligrams)
Branflakes, average serve, 45 g	0.63
Cornflakes, average serve, 40 g	0.58
Muesli, natural, average serve, 60 g	0.70
Muesli, toasted, average serve, 60 g	0.40
Oats, rolled, cooked, average serve, 300 g	0.06
Weetbix, 2 biscuits, 30 g	0.42
Dairy products	
Cheese, average of main varieties, 50 g	0.22
Cheese, cottage, 50 g	0.20
Cheese, ricotta, 50 g	0.10
Cream, average serve, 50 g	0.07
Cream, sour, 1 tablespoon	0.12
Ice cream, 100 mL	0.10
Milk, cow's, regular or skim, 1 cup	0.38
Milk, goat's, 1 cup	0.35
Milk, sheep's, 1 cup	0.80
Soy beverage, 1 cup	0
Soy beverage, fortified, 1 cup	0.48
Yoghurt, fruit, 200 g	0.46
Yoghurt, natural, 200 g	0.76
Meat, poultry and eggs	
Bacon, grilled, 2 rashers, 60 g	0.11
Beef or veal, cooked, average serve, 150 g	0.38
Chicken breast, average serve, 150 g	0.15
Chicken thigh, average serve, 125 g	0.36
Egg, hen, boiled, 1	0.21
Kidney, lamb, cooked, 100 g	1.80
Lamb, cooked, average serve, 150 g	0.36
Liver, cooked, 100 g	4.50
Pork, cooked, average serve, 150 g	0.24
Sausage, grilled, 2	0.22
Fish and seafood	
Crab flesh, cooked, 100 g	0.86
Fish, average fillet, grilled, 200 g	0.40
Mussels, fresh, cooked, 10	0.38

Food	Riboflavin (milligrams)
Mussels, smoked, canned, 6	0.24
Oysters, fresh, 6	0.22
Oysters, smoked, canned, 6	0.23
Salmon, grilled, 200 g	0.28
Salmon, pink or red, canned, 100 g	0.22
Sardines, canned, 100 g	0.20
Tuna, canned, 100 g	0.11
Tuna, fresh, 200 g	0.26
Nuts and seeds	
Almonds, 50 g	0.45
Almonds with skin, 50 g	0.70
Brazil nuts, 50 g	0.22
Cashews, 50 g	0.10
Chestnuts, 50 g	0.01
Coconut	0
Coconut milk, from centre of nut, 1 cup	0.16
Hazelnuts, 50 g	0.09
Macadamias, 50 g	0.05
Peanut butter, 1 tablespoon	0.03
Peanuts, raw with skin, 50 g	0.06
Peanuts, roasted and salted, 50 g	0.08
Pecans, 50 g	0.09
Pine nuts, 50 g	0.10
Pistachios, 50 g	0.15
Pumpkin seeds, 1 tablespoon	0.06
Sesame seeds, 2 teaspoons	0.02
Sunflower seeds, 1 tablespoon	0.04
Tahini paste, 1 tablespoon	0.06
Walnuts, 50 g	0.09
Fruit	
Average piece, fresh	0.02
Banana, 1 medium	0.14
Passionfruit, 2 medium	0.06
Persimmon, 1 medium	0.16

Food	Riboflavin (milligrams)
Vegetables	
Asparagus, steamed, 6 spears	0.10
Avocado, $\frac{1}{2}$ medium	0.15
Beans, broad, cooked, 100 g	0.32
Beans, green, cooked, 100 g	0.09
Broccoli, cooked, average serve, 100 g	0.21
Brussels sprouts, cooked, 6	0.14
Cabbage, green, cooked, 1 cup	0.06
Cabbage, mustard, raw, 1 cup	0.09
Cabbage, red, cooked, 1 cup	0.15
Carrot, mature, cooked, 1 medium	0.06
Carrot, mature, raw, 1 medium	0.06
Cauliflower, cooked, 1 cup	0.15
Chinese greens, cooked, 1 cup	0.10
Endive, raw, average serve, 40 g	0.04
Leek, cooked, $\frac{1}{2}$ cup	0.09
Lettuce, mignonette, 4 leaves	0.04
Lettuce, raddiccio, 4 leaves	0.08
Mushrooms, 100 g	0.40
Okra, cooked, 75 g	0.09
Parsley, $\frac{1}{2}$ cup	0.08
Parsnip, cooked, 1 medium	0.16
Peas, sugar snap or snow, 1 cup	0.08
Peas, green, cooked, 100 g	0.10
Potato, 1 average, 180 g	0.06
Pumpkin, average serve, 120 g	0.10
Silverbeet, cooked, $\frac{1}{2}$ cup	0.12
Spinach, Chinese, raw, 100 g	0.21
Spinach, English, cooked, 100 g	0.15
Sweet corn, baby, 5 spears	0.13
Turnip tops, cooked, $\frac{1}{2}$ cup	0.18
Watercress, raw, 1 cup	0.14
Legumes	
Beans, haricot, cooked, 1 cup	0.10
Beans, kidney, canned, 1 cup	0.09

Food	Riboflavin (milligrams)
Soy beans, cooked, 1 cup	0.11
Tempeh, 50 g	0.24
Take-away foods	
Barbecued chicken, $\frac{1}{4}$	0.12
Big breakfast, 1 serve	0.54
Chiko roll, 1	0.10
Chips, average serve, 150 g	0.05
Fish, battered and fried, 1 piece, 150 g	0.19
Hamburger, 1	0.22
Hamburger, fast food chain, 1	0.56
Hamburger with cheese, 1	0.31
Hamburger with egg, 1	0.42
Meat pie, 1	0.25
Pizza, $\frac{1}{2}$ medium, average, 300 g	0.30
Sausage roll, 1	0.10
Thickshake, 300 mL	0.67
Miscellaneous	
Chocolate, dark, 50 g	0.07
Chocolate, milk, 50 g	0.30
Malted-milk powder, 1 tablespoon	0.54
Marmite, 1 teaspoon	1.05
Ovaltine, 2 teaspoons	0.30
Pasta sauce (tomato based), $\frac{3}{4}$ cup	0.94
Vegemite, 1 teaspoon	1.10

Effect of cooking

Cooking causes some loss of riboflavin. If lemon juice, vinegar or other acid is present, the losses are substantial, so you should squeeze lemon or lime onto foods just before serving. The longer the cooking time and the greater the volume of water, the larger the losses. Adding bicarbonate of soda to vegetables to make them green causes loss of most of the riboflavin. An alternative way to have green vegetables looking bright is to steam them briefly and then plunge them into iced water and drain quickly. To serve them hot, reheat in a microwave or in a pan with a little olive oil. The oil has an added advantage of enhancing absorption of some of the vitamins in the vegetables, especially beta carotene and related carotenoids.

Milk left in sunlight for two hours loses at least 50 per cent of its riboflavin.

Deficiency

It is rare to lack riboflavin without also being deficient in other vitamins and this makes it difficult to pinpoint signs of deficiency. Riboflavin deficiency is not common in countries such as Australia, although it may occur in conjunction with other problems in people with a chronic alcohol problem.

Symptoms may include feeling tired (also occurs with a lack of most other vitamins, iron and sufficient kilojoules) as well as burning itchy eyes and tenderness in the mouth. As the deficiency progresses, there are changes in the skin with dermatitis in the folds around the nose; cheilosis (an area of red denuded skin where the lips close), angular stomatitis (cracks in the corners of the mouth, which can also be caused by dental problems), invasion of the cornea with blood vessels (not visible to the naked eye), conjunctivitis, anaemia and problems with normal brain function.

Riboflavin deficiency can occur as a side effect of other problems that interfere with the way the vitamin is used in the body. These include conditions such as an insufficiency of the thyroid or adrenal glands, and with some drugs used to treat mental illness. Alcohol interferes with the absorption of riboflavin.

A deficiency can be diagnosed from levels in the urine or by measuring one of the enzymes that requires riboflavin.

Excess

It is difficult to assess the effects of excess riboflavin because no more than about 25 milligrams can be absorbed by the body. Even if given intravenously, the vitamin is not very soluble and high levels won't occur. This is probably a natural protective mechanism since excess riboflavin, in theory at least, could damage DNA.

Excessive quantities of riboflavin are not added to many foods because the colour is not considered an incentive for sales. It is, however, added to most processed breakfast cereals, although the quantities are moderate.

Riboflavin supplements

Unless there is a known deficiency of riboflavin, there is no point in taking a supplement. However, people with health problems due to chronic high alcohol consumption need riboflavin supplements. Riboflavin has no effect on hangovers and the appearance of it in urine soon after taking it generally shows that supplements are almost always excess to requirements.

Current research findings

There has been a lot of research to work out all the roles riboflavin has in the body. Now its potential as an antioxidant is exciting some researchers.

There is also research into the possible use of large doses of riboflavin for treating migraine. Researchers in the United States have given 54 people who suffered between two and eight migraines a month either a placebo or 400 milligrams of riboflavin a day. After three months, those taking riboflavin had almost 40 per cent fewer attacks. This study needs to be duplicated with a larger group and some explanation offered for the effect of the vitamin.

NIACIN OR VITAMIN B₃

What it is

Niacin is a generic name for two major compounds that make up this vitamin. They are known as nicotinic acid (no connection with nicotine from tobacco) and nicotinamide.

Nicotinic acid was first isolated in 1867. However, it was not known to be a vitamin until 1937 when researchers showed that a lack of it was the cause of pellagra, a common condition at the time, especially among poor black populations who lived largely on corn. At that time, corn was low in an amino acid called tryptophan, which the body converts into niacin. Corn is now bred to contain much more of this amino acid and pellagra is rarely seen. This was a valuable way to use knowledge about plant breeding.

For many years, nicotinic acid itself was referred to as niacin but once its structure became known, chemists sorted out the differences. For those interested, nicotinic acid is pyridine–3-carboxylic acid and nicotinamide is nicotinic acid amide. Nicotinamide is more soluble in water but either form is rapidly absorbed from the stomach. Both forms attach themselves to complicated molecules and function as essential coenzymes in many of the body's chemical reactions. Nicotinamide is the major form of niacin found in the blood.

Much of the body's niacin is made in the liver from the amino acid tryptophan, although the process slows down if there is a deficiency of vitamin B_6, riboflavin or iron, all of which play a role in the series of chemical reactions needed for the process. The synthesis of compounds that need niacin as a co-factor occurs in all body tissues.

What it does

Niacin is used to make nicotinamide adenine dinucleotide (NAD) and NADP, the form of NAD with a phosphate molecule attached. These compounds are essential for the life of every cell in the body, allowing cells to use energy and DNA to constantly repair themselves from the wear and tear associated with being alive.

Nicotinic acid is involved in the 'glucose tolerance factor', a complex molecule that also contains chromium and is involved in the body's production of insulin. How the vitamin works in this role is not yet known.

Nicotinic acid in large doses can also reduce blood cholesterol levels and levels of triglyceride fats in the blood. This was first reported in 1955, although it was publicised in a popular book published in the 1980s. The dose required is 1500 to 3000 milligrams (1.5–3 grams) a day. Because of its side effects (see *Excess*), it is not commonly recommended for this purpose. Nicotinamide does not have the same effect.

How much you need

Like the other B vitamins discussed so far, the amount of niacin needed depends on energy requirements. The more kilojoules of energy burned, the greater the need for niacin.

Since tryptophan in protein foods also contributes to niacin in the body, the higher the protein content of the diet, the more niacin the body can make for itself. Tryptophan makes up about 1 per cent of the protein in foods and approximately 60 milligrams of tryptophan is needed for the body to make 1 milligram of niacin. In practice, about half the body's niacin comes from the niacin in foods and half comes from tryptophan. These contributions have been taken into account in working out recommended dietary intakes of niacin in various countries. The RDIs may therefore vary in different parts of the world, according to the foods typically consumed.

During the last few months of pregnancy, the amount of tryptophan that is converted to niacin increases by a factor of about three. This effect is caused by oestrogen increasing the enzyme required for the conversion. It is also likely that more tryptophan can be converted to niacin when women take oestrogen in the form of the oral contraceptive pill. This is the reason why women on the pill are often told not to take extra niacin.

The combination of pre-formed niacin and the contribution of niacin from tryptophan is called niacin equivalents (NE). One milligram niacin equivalents = 1 milligram niacin or 60 milligrams tryptophan. You can also calculate niacin equivalents (in milligrams) by adding together the niacin (in milligrams) plus 0.16 times the dietary protein (in grams).

The recommended dietary intake of niacin equivalents is as follows:

Age	RDI (milligrams)
Breast-fed and bottle-fed	4
7–12 months	7
1–3 years	10
4–7 years	12
Boys, 8–11 years	15
Girls, 8–11 years	15
Boys, 12–15 years	20
Girls, 12–15 years	18
Boys, 16–18 years	21
Girls, 16–18 years	16
Men, 19–64 years	19
Men, over 64 years	16
Women, 19–54 years	13
Women, over 54 years	11
Pregnancy	15
Lactation	18

Where it is found

The best sources of niacin include fish (especially tuna), Vegemite, meats (especially liver), wholegrain and fortified cereals, legumes and seeds.

Food	Niacin equivalents (milligrams)
Breads, grains and cereals	
Barley, pearl, cooked, 1 cup, 180 g	3.6
Bran, oat, 1 tablespoon, 15 g	0.6
Bran, rice, 1 tablespoon, 15 g	6.5
Bran, wheat, 1 tablespoon, 8 g	2.1
Bread, multigrain, 1 slice, 30 g	1.1
Bread, white, enriched, 1 slice, 30 g	0.9
Bread, wholemeal, 1 slice, 30 g	1.3

Food	Niacin equivalents (milligrams)
Burghul (cracked wheat), soaked, $\frac{1}{2}$ cup, 100 g	4.1
Cornmeal, coarse, 1 cup, 200 g	5.6
Flour, white, 1 cup, 125 g	1.4
Flour, wholemeal, 1 cup, 130 g	9.8
Millet flour, 1 cup, 130 g	5.0
Muffin, English, toasted, 1, 60 g	2.2
Oats, rolled, raw, $\frac{1}{2}$ cup, 50 g	1.9
Pasta, cooked, 1 cup, 180 g	2.2
Pasta, egg noodles, cooked, 1 cup, 180 g	2.3
Pasta, wholemeal, cooked, 1 cup, 180 g	4.7
Rice, brown, cooked, 1 cup, 180 g	4.3
Rice, sungold, cooked, 1 cup, 180 g	4.0
Rice, white, cooked, 1 cup, 180 g	2.2
Rye flour, 1 cup, 130 g	4.8
Wheat germ, 1 tablespoon, 10 g	1.0
Breakfast cereals	
Allbran, $\frac{1}{2}$ cup, 40 g	6.4
Branflakes, average serve, 45 g	8.5
Cornflakes, average serve, 40 g	4.3
Muesli, natural, average serve, 60 g	7.6
Muesli, toasted, average serve, 60 g	3.5
Oats, rolled, cooked, average serve, 300 g	0.9
Semolina, cooked, 1 cup, 180 g	0.9
Weetbix, 2 biscuits, 30 g	2.5
Dairy products	
Cheese, average of main varieties, 50 g	2.3
Milk, cow's, regular or skim, 1 cup	1.5
Milk, goat's, 1 cup	2.5
Milk, sheep's, 1 cup	2.6
Soy beverage, fortified, 250 mL	3.4
Soy beverage, unfortified, 250 mL	2.5
Yoghurt, natural, 200 g	2.0
Yoghurt, fruit, 200 g	1.4

Food	Niacin equivalents (milligrams)
Meat, poultry and eggs	
Bacon, grilled, 2 rashers, 60 g	8.0
Beef, veal, lamb or pork, cooked, 150 g	17.0
Chicken, cooked, $\frac{1}{4}$ medium	18.0
Egg, hen, boiled, 1	1.0
Kidney, lamb, 100 g	13.5
Liver, cooked, 100 g	19.0
Sausages, grilled, 2	8.0
Fish and seafood	
Crab flesh, cooked, 100 g	10.2
Fish, white, grilled, average fillet, 200 g	18.5
Mussels, 10	5.0
Octopus, 100 g	8.8
Prawns, cooked, 6 medium	6.8
Salmon, grilled, 200 g	24.5
Salmon, pink or red, canned, 100 g	7.3
Sardines, canned, 100 g	11.7
Tuna, fresh, 200 g	34.5
Nuts and seeds	
Almonds, 50 g	3.6
Brazil nuts, 50 g	1.5
Cashews, 50 g	3.7
Chestnuts, 50 g	0.5
Coconut, fresh, 50 g	0.6
Hazelnuts, 50 g	2.3
Macadamias, 50 g	1.7
Peanut butter, 1 tablespoon	5.6
Peanuts, 50 g	11.4
Pecans, 50 g	1.5
Pine nuts, 50 g	3.3
Pistachios, 50 g	2.4
Pumpkin seeds, 1 tablespoon	4.4

Food	Niacin equivalents (milligrams)
Sesame seeds, 2 teaspoons	0.9
Sunflower seeds, 1 tablespoon	3.7
Tahini paste, 1 tablespoon	2.4
Walnuts, 50 g	1.9
Fruit	
Average piece, fresh	0.8
Passionfruit, 2 medium	1.5
Sultanas or raisins, 50 g	0.08
Vegetables	
Artichoke, globe, cooked, 1	0.5
Asparagus, steamed, 6 spears	0.8
Avocado, $\frac{1}{2}$ medium	2.5
Beans, broad, cooked, 100 g	3.1
Beans, green, cooked, 100 g	0.8
Broccoli, cooked, average serve, 100 g	1.2
Brussels sprouts, cooked, 6	1.1
Cabbage, green or red, cooked, 1 cup	0.6
Capsicum, green, raw, $\frac{1}{2}$ medium	1.0
Capsicum, red, raw, $\frac{1}{2}$ medium	1.5
Carrot, mature, raw or cooked, 1 medium	1.2
Cassava, boiled, 100 g	0.8
Cauliflower, cooked, 1 cup	1.0
Celeriac, cooked, 100 g	1.1
Chilli, red, 1 small	0.4
Eggplant, cooked, 1 slice, 100 g	0.9
Mushrooms, 100 g	4.1
Okra, cooked, 100 g	1.7
Onion, 1 medium	1.0
Spring onion, each	0.4
Parsley, $\frac{1}{2}$ cup	0.3
Parsnip, cooked, 1 medium	1.9
Pea, sugar snap or snow, 100 g	1.4
Peas, green, cooked, 100 g	2.5

Food	Niacin equivalents (milligrams)
Potato, average serve, 180 g	3.2
Pumpkin, Queensland blue, average serve, 120 g	1.3
Salad, green, average serve	0.8
Spinach, English, cooked, 100 g	1.1
Spinach, Chinese, raw, 100 g	1.3
Squash, scallopini, cooked, 3	0.8
Sweet potato, average serve, 150 g	1.5
Sweet corn, canned, $\frac{1}{2}$ cup	2.0
Sweet corn, cooked, 1 cob	2.9
Tomato, 1 medium, 150 g	1.2
Tomatoes, egg, 2 medium, 150 g	1.5
Turnip, cooked, 100 g	1.0
Watercress, 50 g	0.7
Zucchini, cooked, 1 medium	1.0
Legumes	
Baked beans, canned, 1 cup	3.2
Beans, haricot, cooked, 1 cup	3.7
Beans, kidney, cooked or canned, 1 cup	2.9
Chickpeas, cooked or canned, 1 cup	3.0
Lentils, cooked, 1 cup	3.2
Split peas, cooked, 1 cup	2.9
Soy beans, cooked, 1 cup	8.6
Take-away foods	
Barbecued chicken, $\frac{1}{4}$	10.9
Big breakfast, 1 serve	8.6
Chiko roll, 1	3.9
Chips, average serve, 150 g	3.0
Corn chips, 50 g	1.3
Fish, battered and fried, 1 piece, 150 g	12.0
Garlic bread, 2 slices	0.9
Hamburger, 1	6.4
Hamburger, fast food chain, 1	13.0
Hamburger with egg, 1	8.3

Food	Niacin equivalents (milligrams)
Meat pie, 1	9.0
Pizza, $\frac{1}{2}$ medium, average 300 g	12.0
Potato crisps, 50 g	2.4
Pretzels, 50 g	1.3
Sausage roll, 1	4.3
Thickshake, chocolate, 300 mL	2.7
Drinks	
Apple juice, 250 mL	1.9
Coffee, black, 150 mL	1.4
Cappuccino, average cup	1.5
Grape juice, dark, 250 mL	2.8
Orange juice, 250 mL	1.8
Pineapple juice, 250 mL	2.3
Tomato juice 250 mL	1.8
Miscellaneous	
Bonox, 1 teaspoon	0.01
Chocolate, 50 g	0.06
Malted-milk powder, 1 tablespoon	0.44
Marmite, 1 teaspoon	0.55
Muesli bar, 1, 60 g	0.07
Ovaltine, 2 teaspoons	0.31
Vegemite, 1 teaspoon	0.90

Effect of cooking

Niacin is present in uncooked foods as the dinucleotides NAD and NADP, although in cereals it may be linked with amino acids and certain natural sugars. In traditional varieties of corn, the niacin is bound in a form that makes it unusable unless the corn is first soaked in lime water. This was a common custom in Central America before corn was ground to make tortillas and the soaking is still practised in some areas. Newer varieties of corn have more niacin and higher levels of tryptophan, so the pre-soaking is less necessary.

Deficiency

A deficiency of niacin is not seen in developed countries and pellagra—the classic deficiency disease—is now seen only in countries where there is chronic starvation and gross malnutrition. It is usually accompanied by a lack of most other nutrients and some of the symptoms may be due to associated deficiency of riboflavin.

Before pellagra occurs, a deficiency of niacin causes changes in the skin with a pigmented rash occurring symmetrically in areas of the body exposed to sunlight. The tongue may also become bright red and changes may occur in the intestinal tract, accompanied by vomiting, diarrhoea or constipation. Depression, tiredness, headache and apathy also develop and then memory loss becomes common. However, the memory loss in conditions such as Alzheimer's disease is not due to niacin deficiency.

Some drugs may also cause a niacin deficiency by interfering with the conversion of tryptophan to niacin. Isoniazid, a prescription drug used to treat tuberculosis, can have this effect and should be taken with a supplement of niacin (and also vitamin B_6 to avoid some other interactions).

Few people in developed countries will have niacin deficiency. Measuring niacin levels in blood plasma does not give an indication of niacin status. The best test for niacin deficiency is probably to measure the level of nicotinamide adenine dinucleotide (NAD) in blood cells known as erythrocytes.

Excess

Large doses (1500 to 3000 milligrams [1.5–3 grams] a day) of nicotinic acid taken to reduce blood cholesterol cause hot flushes, similar to those experienced by women during menopause. However, the nicotinic acid not only produces feelings of heat and makes the skin turn red (looking like a bad case of sunburn), it may also cause skin rashes and increase uric acid levels, leading to gout in susceptible people. It can also cause liver problems and abnormalities in the eyes. Some people taking high doses of nicotinic acid also develop high levels of sugar in the blood. All the effects disappear once the high dose is discontinued, but they are good reasons to use other methods of reducing high levels of blood cholesterol.

Nicotinamide does not have any effect on blood cholesterol levels, so there is no reason to take a high dose. Rats given high doses of nicotinamide do not grow and they also develop fatty liver. For these reasons, high doses of this vitamin are not recommended for human trials.

Niacin supplements

After the publicity given to Daniel Kowalski's book, *The 8-week cholesterol cure* in 1987, many people started taking niacin (as nicotinic acid) to reduce their blood cholesterol levels. Kowalski also recommended large quantities of oat bran, although he wrote that even without dietary changes, niacin would reduce blood cholesterol. There is plenty of medical evidence to back such claims.

However, because of the side effects that nicotinic acid can cause, it should not be used unless you have had tests of liver function and also established that you do not have high uric acid levels. Those with diabetes, gastric ulcers, gout or any abnormalities in the liver should avoid it. As heavy alcohol consumption stresses the liver, it is almost certainly not a good idea for big drinkers to take nicotinic acid.

Most people can reduce blood cholesterol levels by decreasing saturated fats in the diet. This is a better method. If you decide to try nicotinic acid tablets, including slow-release varieties that are supposed to reduce flushing, it is important to have your doctor check your liver and uric acid levels regularly.

Current research findings

Smaller doses of nicotinamide of up to 1500 milligrams (1.5 grams) a day are being trialled for people with insulin-dependent diabetes. At this stage, there are no conclusive results that it is of benefit.

PANTOTHENIC ACID

What it is

Once known as vitamin B_5, pantothenic acid is sometimes referred to as pantothenate. Pantothen is a Greek word meaning 'from all sides'. This reflects the ubiquitous nature of pantothenic acid, which occurs in all living matter. The vitamin is found in almost all foods and takes part in many thousands of biochemical reactions within the body.

Pantothenic acid was first discovered in 1933 as an essential factor for yeast. It was isolated in 1939 as the factor that would prevent dermatitis in chickens and stop black hair turning grey in rats. Its significance for humans was not really established until 1947 when researchers found that it is the main constituent of coenzyme A. Usually written as CoA, this enzyme takes part in many thousands of chemical reactions within the body. (A coenzyme is the non-protein part of an enzyme which forms a loose association with a protein component to make up the complete enzyme.)

When isolated, pantothenic acid is a pale yellow oily liquid, possibly showing its relationship to the fact that it is a derivative of butyric acid—a fatty acid found in butter. The calcium or sodium salts of pantothenic acid will form a crystalline structure that can be used in supplements. Supplements also contain panthenol, an alcohol derivative of pantothenic acid.

What it does

Although the hair of rats fed a diet deficient in pantothenic acid goes grey, there is no evidence that pantothenic acid has any role in greying of human hair. Nor is there any evidence that taking extra pantothenic acid can stop human hair losing its colour with age.

Pantothenic acid has different roles in various animal species. In humans, as part of CoA, it is involved in the way the body makes fatty acids and uses them for energy and as central components of all cell membranes and nerve cells. Pantothenic acid is involved in most of the body's biochemistry and there is no doubt we could not survive without it. Some of its many functions involve the body's synthesis of several amino acids that make up protein, as well as being involved in making cholesterol, sex hormones, vitamins A, D and B_{12}, and porphyrin (which is then used to make haemoglobin).

The true essentiality of pantothenic acid was only

recognised in the 1950s and '60s when researchers deliberately gave humans a diet containing a substance that would antagonise the action of pantothenic acid. Without the vitamin, the subjects developed many symptoms (see *Deficiency*).

How much you need

No formal recommended dietary intake has been set for pantothenic acid because natural deficiencies cannot be found and no one wants to repeat the early experiments of making people deficient in the vitamin in order to find out how much is needed. However, experimental work has led to an estimate of 4 to 7 milligrams a day for adults, 2 milligrams a day for infants and 4 to 5 milligrams a day for children seven to ten years of age. One study of teenagers found that even those on a poor diet and getting less than 4 milligrams a day had normal concentrations of pantothenic acid in the blood. They were also excreting normal quantities of pantothenic acid in the urine. The true requirements may therefore be a little lower than the usual recommendations.

Bacteria living in the intestine can also make pantothenic acid, although no one knows how much of this can be absorbed.

Where it is found

Most human diets provide between 5 and 20 milligrams of pantothenic acid a day, easily meeting the estimated requirements. Almost all foods contain pantothenic acid. Royal jelly contains pantothenic acid, produced by worker bees for their queen. As royal jelly can cause severe, even life-threatening allergic reactions in some humans, it makes more sense to get the vitamin from foods. If a high intake was desired (although there are no known benefits) fish roe is a much richer and safer source than royal jelly.

The best food sources include fish roe, kidney, liver, salmon, prawns, poultry, egg yolk, peanuts, milk, yoghurt and meat (especially pork). Breast milk is high in this vitamin and the content increases five-fold after four days.

Food	Pantothenic acid (milligrams)
Breads, grains and cereals	
Barley, wholegrain, cooked, 1 cup, 180 g	1.3
Bran, wheat, 1 tablespoon, 8 g	0.2
Bread, multigrain, 1 slice, 30 g	0.1
Bread, white, 1 slice, 30 g	0.1
Bread, wholemeal or rye, 1 slice, 30 g	0.2
Flour, white, 1 cup, 125 g	0.5
Flour, wholemeal, 1 cup, 130 g	1.0
Oats, rolled, raw, $\frac{1}{2}$ cup, 50 g	0.5
Pasta, wholemeal, cooked, 1 cup, 180 g	0.4
Rice, white, cooked, 1 cup, 180 g	0.4
Rye flour, 1 cup, 130 g	1.3
Soy flour, 1 cup, 150 g	2.4
Wheat germ, 1 tablespoon, 10 g	0.2
Breakfast cereals	
Bran cereals, average serve, $\frac{1}{2}$ cup, 40 g	0.7
Branflakes, average serve, 45 g	0.4
Cornflakes, average serve, 40 g	0.1
Muesli, natural, average serve, 60 g	0.7
Oats, rolled, cooked, average serve, 300 g	0.6
Wheat breakfast biscuits, 2, 30 g	0.2
Dairy products	
Cheese, average of main varieties, 50 g	0.2

Food	Pantothenic acid (milligrams)
Cheese, Stilton, 50 g	0.4
Ice cream, 2 scoops, 100 g	0.4
Milk, cow's, 1 cup	0.9
Milk, goat's, 1 cup	1.0
Milk, sheep's, 1 cup	1.1
Milk, skim, 1 cup	0.8
Yoghurt, fruit, 200 g	0.6
Yoghurt, natural, regular or low-fat, 200 g	1.0
Meat, poultry and eggs	
Bacon, grilled, 2 rashers, 60 g	0.4
Beef or veal, cooked, average serve, 150 g	1.2
Chicken, cooked, $\frac{1}{4}$ medium	1.8
Duck, cooked, 150 g	2.3
Egg, hen, boiled, 1	0.9
Fish, grilled, average fillet, 200 g	0.7
Kidney, lamb, 100 g	7.7
Lamb, cooked, average serve, 150 g	1.1
Liver, cooked, 100 g	11.0
Pâté, 50 g	1.1
Pork, cooked, average serve, 150 g	1.8
Prawns, cooked, 6 medium	1.4
Roe, 1 teaspoon	11.6
Salmon, grilled, 200 g	3.6
Salmon, pink or red, canned, 100 g	0.5
Sardines, canned, 100 g	0.5
Turkey, roast, 150 g	1.2
Nuts and seeds	
Almonds, 50 g	0.2
Brazil nuts, 50 g	0.2
Cashews, 50 g	0.5
Chestnuts, 50 g	0.3
Coconut, fresh, 50 g	0.2
Hazelnuts, 50 g	0.8
Macadamias, 50 g	0.3

Food	Pantothenic acid (milligrams)
Peanut butter, 1 tablespoon	0.4
Peanuts, raw with skin, 50 g	1.3
Peanuts, roasted and salted, 50 g	0.9
Pecans, 50 g	0.9
Sesame seeds, 2 teaspoons	0.2
Tahini paste, 1 tablespoon	0.6
Walnuts, 50 g	0.8
Fruit	
Apple, 1 average	trace
Apricots, 2 average	0.3
Apricots, dried, 6	0.4
Avocado, $\frac{1}{2}$ medium	0.5
Banana, 1 average	0.4
Blackberries and other berries, 100 g	0.3
Cherries, 200 g	0.4
Custard apple, 150 g	0.4
Dates, dried, 6	0.4
Grapefruit, $\frac{1}{2}$ medium	0.4
Grapes, 200 g	0.1
Mango, 1 average	0.2
Melon, 200g slice	0.3
Orange, 1 medium	0.5
Peach, 1 average	0.2
Pear, 1 medium	0.1
Pomegranate, 100 g	0.6
Prunes, 6	0.2
Raisins or sultanas, 50 g	0.1
Strawberries, $\frac{1}{2}$ punnet, 125 g	0.4
Vegetables	
Asparagus, steamed, 6 spears	0.1
Beans, broad, cooked, 100 g	3.8
Beans, green, cooked, 100 g	0.1
Broccoli, cooked, average serve, 100 g	0.7
Brussels sprouts, cooked, 6	0.3

Food	Pantothenic acid (milligrams)
Cabbage, green, cooked, 1 cup	0.2
Capsicum, green or red, raw, $\frac{1}{2}$ medium	0.1
Carrot, mature, cooked, 1 medium	0.2
Carrot, mature, raw, 1 medium	0.3
Cauliflower, cooked, 1 cup	0.4
Celery, raw, 100 g	0.4
Chinese greens, 100 g	0.4
Cucumber, 100 g	0.3
Lettuce, 2 leaves	0.1
Mushrooms, cooked, 100 g	1.4
Mushrooms, raw, 100 g	2.0
Onion, cooked, 100 g	0.2
Parsnip, 100 g	0.4
Parsley, $\frac{1}{2}$ cup	0.1
Peas, green, cooked, 100 g	0.1
Potato, 1 average, 200 g	0.8
Pumpkin, average serve, 120 g	0.4
Snow peas, cooked, 100 g	0.7
Spinach, English, cooked, 100g	0.2
Sweet corn, canned, 100 g	0.2
Sweet corn, cooked, 1 cob	0.6
Sweet potato, average serve, 150 g	0.8
Tomato, 1 medium, 150 g	0.4
Zucchini, cooked, 1 average	0.1
Legumes	
Baked beans, canned, 1 cup	0.4
Beans, black eye, cooked, 1 cup	0.6
Beans, haricot, cooked, 1 cup	0.4
Beans, kidney, canned, 1 cup	0.3
Chickpeas, cooked, 1 cup	0.6
Lentils, cooked, 1 cup	0.6
Soy beans, cooked, 1 cup	0.4
Split peas, cooked, 1 cup	0.6
Tofu, 100 g	0.1

Food	Pantothenic acid (milligrams)
Miscellaneous	
Beer, bitter, 250 mL	25.0
Beer, premium lager, 250 mL	0.1
Chocolate, 50 g	0.3
Potato crisps, 50 g	0.4
Pretzels, 50 g	0.1
Royal jelly, 1 g	0.5
Stout, 250 mL	0.1
Tea, 1 cup, 200 mL	0.1
Yeast, dried, 2 teaspoons	1.1

Effect of cooking

Some pantothenic acid is lost in cooking, with losses of 15 to 50 per cent of the original levels being common. Canning causes even greater losses.

Deficiency

A deficiency of pantothenic acid is rare in humans and only occurs in cases of severe malnutrition, along with deficiencies of almost every nutrient. Experimentally, a deficiency has been induced by giving volunteers a compound which interferes with the action of pantothenic acid. Under such circumstances, symptoms included apathy, abdominal pains, vomiting, inability to sleep, fatigue, cramps in the legs and 'pins and needles' in fingers and toes. An increased sensitivity to insulin and a fall in the white blood cell count also occurred.

Many people get cramps in the legs and 'pins and needles' in fingers and toes. Some brochures for pantothenic acid supplements suggest that this is due to a deficiency. However, cramps are often due to slight dehydration, and 'pins and needles' come from poor circulation. Neither of these symptoms is ordinarily due to a lack of pantothenic acid and there is no evidence that taking supplements or using royal jelly will have any effect.

Deficiency of pantothenic acid has different effects in various species of animals but these cannot be extrapolated to humans. For example, black rats develop grey hair but also the adrenal cortex of the kidney shrinks and they begin to haemorrhage. As well, they show increased resistance to some viruses. Chickens develop dermatitis, dogs become hypoglycaemic, their heart rate increases and they can develop convulsions, and monkeys become anaemic.

Excess

The vitamin appears to be non-toxic although huge doses of 10 000 to 20 000 milligrams can produce diarrhoea. Mice die when given a dose of 10 milligrams per kilogram of body weight.

Pantothenic acid supplements

There is no evidence that supplements of pantothenic acid are of any use except in cases of severe malnutrition, when the vitamin should be given, along with every other vitamin. In spite of the popularity of royal jelly, there is no evidence that it has any benefits. People who take or sell royal jelly often claim that it is a 'super supplement' or 'wonder food', but they do not have any evidence apart from their personal opinion to back such claims. In Australia, royal jelly must now carry a statement warning about the possible harmful allergic reactions it can cause. Health authorities took this decision when a person with asthma died after consuming royal jelly.

There have been mixed results when giving athletes a supplement of pantothenic acid. One study reported that highly trained endurance athletes given 2000 milligrams a day for two weeks had decreased levels of lactic acid (which causes fatigue) and decreased their oxygen consumption. However, another well-controlled study using 1000 milligrams a day for two weeks in highly trained distance runners found no difference in performance or blood levels of any standard parameters.

Current research findings

Animals made deficient in pantothenic acid develop a condition not unlike ulcerative colitis. Some researchers have therefore theorised that levels of pantothenic acid may be low within the lining of the large bowel in human cases of ulcerative colitis. At this stage, they do not have evidence that extra pantothenic acid will help in this condition. Current studies are still elucidating the way that pantothenic acid and CoA work in fixing particular fatty acids in cell membranes. This work is intensely complicated biochemistry and is being done to establish biochemical pathways. There is no suggestion that humans may benefit from more or less pantothenic acid than is present in the average diet.

PYRIDOXINE OR VITAMIN B$_6$

What it is

Like many of the vitamins in the B complex, pyridoxine is actually a group of substances with three members—pyridoxine, pyridoxal and pyridoxamine. First discovered in 1934, the vitamin was synthesised in 1936, although research continues into all its functions. Each of the three forms of the vitamin are interconverted within the body and each functions as a coenzyme to help various enzymes carry out multiple roles within the body. The vitamin is carried in the blood in both plasma and in red cells and is taken up by the liver where it is converted to its most active form—pyridoxal 5-phosphate. About 80 to 90 per cent of the body's B_6 is stored in muscles.

What it does

There are about 100 enzymes in the body that need vitamin B_6. Its known roles include a part in the process gluconeogenesis, in which glucose is produced from amino acids. This process is especially important during exercise. If intake of vitamin B_6 is low, there is no effect on blood sugar levels but there can be an adverse effect on glucose tolerance. This means that without enough B_6, the body is unable to adapt well to changing levels of glucose within the blood, probably because the secretion of insulin is not functioning normally.

The nervous system also relies heavily on vitamin B_6 and it is especially important during pregnancy. Infants given a formula milk which had lost its vitamin B_6 due to overheating of the formula developed abnormal electroencephalogram (EEG) patterns. There is also an increased risk of convulsions. Studies in rats to trace what is happening in such circumstances show that vitamin B_6 deficiency in a mother rat leads to altered levels of long-chain fatty acids in the brain of her offspring. Some of the signs of depression and other mental disorders seen when there is a deficiency of vitamin B_6 also point to the vitamin's involvement in the transmission of nerve impulses.

Vitamin B_6 is involved in fat metabolism, although all its effects are not yet understood. In rats, a deficiency of vitamin B_6 leads to a decreased level of body fat and lower levels of fats in the blood. However, a deficiency of vitamin B_6 in humans is not associated with any reduction in blood cholesterol levels.

One of the most important functions of vitamin B_6 involves the immune system. This is a balancing act in that low levels of B_6 adversely affect some aspects of immunity, whereas high levels may have undesirable effects on the growth of some tumours. The active form of vitamin B_6, pyridoxal 5-phosphate, may be a good defence against viruses, possibly by having an effect on DNA synthesis. However, this does not mean that more is better.

When the amino acid tryptophan is being converted to niacin (see *Niacin*), vitamin B_6 is also needed. The reaction can still proceed in people who have a low intake of B_6, but it is less efficient and the amount of niacin produced is slightly reduced. However, the lowered production of niacin may explain the dermatitis and skin changes seen with gross deficiency of vitamin B_6.

To add to its string of reactions within the body, researchers have now shown that vitamin B_6 can modulate the action of the body's steroid hormones. The vitamin can bind to steroid receptors, thus displacing the effects of high levels of hormones such as oestrogen, which can be related to cancers of the breast and endometrium. This is a little like what happens with phytoestrogens from plants, although the mechanism may not necessarily be the same. When doses of oral contraceptive pills contained larger doses of oestrogen, it was known that women taking these pills required extra quantities of vitamin B_6. This is no longer relevant with the lower doses of oestrogen in the pill these days but some literature accompanying B_6 supplements may still quote it.

How much you need

The Australian National Health and Medical Research Council has calculated requirements for vitamin B_6, based on an amount of 0.02 milligrams of the vitamin for every gram of protein consumed. (Some countries work on a basis of 0.016 milligrams of B_6 for each gram of protein.) Average protein requirements have been included in the estimate, and a safety margin of 33 per cent has been added. The estimation for lactation has been based on the quantity present in human milk, plus the mother's own needs.

The recommended dietary intake of vitamin B_6 is as follows:

Age	RDI (milligrams)
Breast-fed and bottle-fed	0.25
7–12 months	0.45
1–3 years	0.6–0.9
4–7 years	0.8–1.3
Boys, 8–11 years	1.1–1.6
Girls, 8–11 years	1.0–1.5
Boys, 12–15 years	1.4–2.1
Girls, 12–15 years	1.2–1.8
Boys, 16–18 years	1.5–2.2
Girls, 16–18 years	1.1–1.6
Men, 19–64 years	1.3–1.9

Age	RDI (milligrams)
Men, over 64 years	1.0–1.5
Women, 19–54 years	0.9–1.4
Women, over 54 years	0.8–1.1
Pregnancy	1.0–1.5
Lactation	1.6–2.2

In some other countries, the adult recommendation is 2.0 milligrams a day for males over 15 years of age and 1.6 milligrams for females over 19 years of age, with levels of 2.2 milligrams recommended for pregnancy and 2.1 milligrams for lactation.

Where it is found

In animal foods, vitamin B_6 occurs mainly as pyridoxal or its phosphorylated form. (This helps to trap the B_6 into a stable form and the process occurs in foods and within the body.) In vegetable foods, more of the B_6 is present as pyridoxine and pyridoxamine (or their phosphorylated forms). Some foods, such as rice bran, also contain vitamin B_6 as glycosylated pyridoxine which is less well absorbed.

Good food sources include wheat germ, some breakfast cereals, meats, especially pork, and fish, peanuts, avocadoes, potatoes and legumes.

Food	Vitamin B_6 content (milligrams)
Breads, grains and cereals	
Barley, wholegrain, $\frac{1}{4}$ cup, raw, 45 g	0.25
Bran, wheat, 1 tablespoon, 8 g	0.25
Bread, white, 1 slice, 30 g	0.02

Food	Vitamin B$_6$ content (milligrams)
Bread, wholemeal, 1 slice, 30 g	0.04
Buckwheat, $\frac{1}{2}$ cup raw, 80 g	0.32
Flour, white, 1 cup, 125 g	0.19
Flour, wholemeal, 1 cup, 130 g	0.39
Oats, rolled, raw, $\frac{1}{2}$ cup, 50 g	0.16
Pasta, egg noodles, cooked, 1 cup, 180 g	0.02
Pasta, white, cooked, 1 cup, 180 g	0.04
Pasta, wholemeal, cooked, 1 cup, 180 g	0.14
Rice, white, cooked, 1 cup, 180 g	0.09
Rye flour, 1 cup, 130 g	0.46
Soy flour, low-fat, 1 cup, 150 g	0.78
Wheat germ, 1 tablespoon, 10 g	0.33
Breakfast cereals	
Allbran, $\frac{1}{2}$ cup, 40 g	0.72*
Branflakes, average serve, 45 g	0.81*
Cornflakes, average serve, 40 g	0.71*
Muesli, natural, average serve, 60 g	0.96*
Oats, rolled, cooked, average serve, 300 g	0.12
Weetbix, 2 biscuits, 30 g	0.07*
Dairy products	
Cheese, average of main varieties, 50 g	0.06
Cheese, cottage, 50 g	0.04
Cheese, ricotta, 50 g	0.01
Cheese, soy, 50 g	0.10
Cream, regular or sour, 50 g	0.02
Fromage frais, fruit flavoured, 150 g	0.06
Ice cream, 100 mL	0.05
Milk, cow's, regular or skim, 1 cup	0.15
Milk, goat's, 1 cup	0.15
Milk, sheep's, 1 cup	0.20
Yoghurt, fruit, regular or low-fat, 200 g	0.14
Yoghurt, natural, regular or low-fat, 200 g	0.20

* Values are for UK products

Food	Vitamin B$_6$ content (milligrams)
Meat, poultry and eggs	
Bacon, grilled, 2 rashers, 60 g	0.16
Beef or veal, cooked, average serve, 150 g	0.44
Chicken breast, average serve, 150 g	0.40
Chicken thigh, average serve, 125 g	0.28
Duck, average serve, 150 g	0.37
Egg, hen, boiled, 1	0.07
Egg, duck, 1 average	0.20
Kidney, lamb, cooked, 100 g	0.30
Lamb, cooked, average serve, 150 g	0.36
Liver, cooked, 100 g	0.48
Pork, cooked, average serve, 150 g	0.60
Rabbit, cooked, average serve, 150 g	0.39
Sausages, grilled, 2	0.10
Fish and seafood	
Crab flesh, cooked, 100 g	0.16
Fish, grilled, average fillet, 200 g	0.48
Mussels, fresh, cooked, 10	0.10
Oysters, fresh, 6	0.14
Salmon, grilled, 200 g	1.62
Salmon, pink or red, canned, 100 g	0.21
Sardines, canned, 100 g	0.18
Tuna, canned, 100 g	0.50
Tuna, fresh, 200 g	0.76
Nuts and seeds	
Almonds, 50 g	0.08
Brazil nuts, 50 g	0.16
Cashews, 50 g	0.25
Chestnuts, 50 g	0.17
Coconut, fresh, 50 g	0.03
Coconut milk, from centre of nut, 1 cup	0.08
Hazelnuts, 50 g	0.30

Food	Vitamin B$_6$ content (milligrams)
Macadamias, 50 g	0.14
Peanut butter, 1 tablespoon	0.16
Peanuts, roasted and salted, 50 g	0.32
Pecans, 50 g	0.10
Pine nuts, 50 g	0.17
Pistachios, 50 g	0.17
Pumpkin seeds, 1 tablespoon	0.01
Sesame seeds, 2 teaspoons	0.08
Sunflower seeds, 1 tablespoon	0.02
Tahini paste, 1 tablespoon	0.21
Walnuts, 50 g	0.34
Fruit	
Apple, 1 average	0.12
Apricots, 2 average	0.14
Apricots, dried, 6	0.10
Avocado, $\frac{1}{2}$ medium	0.36
Banana, 1 average	0.65
Blackberries and other berries, 100 g	0.06
Cherries, 200 g	0.10
Dates, dried, 6	0.07
Figs, dried, 50 g	0.09
Grapefruit, $\frac{1}{2}$ medium	0.04
Grapes, 200 g	0.20
Kiwi fruit, 1 average	0.15
Mango, 1 average	0.18
Melon, 200 g slice	0.20
Orange, 1 medium	0.20
Peach, 1 average	0.02
Pear, 1 medium	0.06
Pomegranate, 100 g	0.31
Prunes, 6	0.20
Raisins or sultanas, 50 g	0.13
Strawberries, $\frac{1}{2}$ punnet, 125 g	0.08

Food	Vitamin B$_6$ content (milligrams)
Tamarillo, 1 medium	0.18
Vegetables	
Artichoke, globe, cooked, 100 g	0.08
Asparagus, steamed, 6 spears	0.03
Beans, broad, cooked, 100 g	0.08
Beans, green, cooked, 100 g	0.06
Bean sprouts, 1 cup, 100 g	0.08
Broccoli, cooked, average serve, 100 g	0.11
Brussels sprouts, cooked, 6	0.19
Cabbage, green, cooked, 1 cup	0.08
Cabbage, green, raw, 1 cup, 90 g	0.15
Cabbage, red, cooked, 1 cup	0.05
Capsicum, green, raw, 100 g	0.30
Capsicum, red, raw, 100 g	0.36
Carrot, mature, cooked, 1 medium	0.12
Cauliflower, cooked, 1 cup	0.15
Chinese greens, cooked, 1 cup	0.11
Endive, raw, average serve, 40 g	0.01
Fennel, raw, 100 g	0.06
Kale, cooked, 100 g	0.13
Leek, cooked, $\frac{1}{2}$ cup	0.05
Lettuce, 4 leaves	0.04
Mushrooms, fried, 100 g	0.19
Okra, cooked, 75 g	0.15
Onion, baked, 1 medium	0.38
Parsley, $\frac{1}{2}$ cup	0.02
Parsnip, cooked, 1 medium	0.10
Peas, sugar snap or snow, 100 g	0.18
Peas, green, cooked, $\frac{1}{2}$ cup	0.11
Potato, cooked, 1 average, 180 g	0.59
Pumpkin, average serve, 120 g	0.04
Silverbeet, cooked, $\frac{1}{2}$ cup	0.19
Spinach, English, cooked, 100 g	0.09

Food	Vitamin B$_6$ content (milligrams)
Spinach, English, raw, 100 g	0.17
Sweet corn kernels, 1 cup	0.22
Sweet potato, cooked, 150 g	0.10
Tomato, raw, 1 medium, 150 g	0.21
Tomato puree, $\frac{1}{2}$ cup	0.55
Watercress, raw, 1 cup	0.12
Legumes	
Beans, baked, 1 cup	0.19
Beans, haricot, cooked, 1 cup	0.30
Beans, kidney, canned, 1 cup	0.19
Chickpeas, cooked, 1 cup	0.24
Lentils, cooked, 1 cup	0.39
Soy beans, cooked, 1 cup	0.41
Fats and oils	
All types	0
Take-away foods	
Barbecued chicken, $\frac{1}{4}$	0.56
Chicken, fried, 2 pieces	0.48
Chips, average serve, 150 g	0.40
Fish, battered and fried, 1 piece, 150 g	0.40
Hamburger, 1	0.19
Hamburger, fast food chain, 1	0.32
Hamburger with cheese or egg, 1	0.23
Meat pie, 1	0.12
Milkshake, 1 average	0.08
Pizza, $\frac{1}{2}$ medium, average, 300 g	0.36
Sausage roll, 1	0.09
Miscellaneous	
Beer, premium lager or bitter, 250 mL	0.18
Beer, stout, 250 mL	0.20
Blackcurrant juice drink, 20 mL	0.02
Chocolate, milk, 50 g	0.02

Food	Vitamin B$_6$ content (milligrams)
Fish sauce, 1 tablespoon	0.08
Liquorice, 50 g	0.28
Marmite, 1 teaspoon	0.05
Pasta sauce (tomato based), $\frac{3}{4}$ cup	0.24
Peanut brittle, 50 g	0.10
Potato crisps, 50 g	0.40
Soy beverage, 1 cup	0.18
Tempeh, 50 g	0.15–0.93
Yeast, dried, 2 teaspoons	0.20
Yeast extract, 1 teaspoon	0.08

Effect of cooking

Food processing, storage and cooking all affect vitamin B$_6$ in some foods. Losses of 10 to 50 per cent can occur during processing and heating. Even greater losses occur in cooking foods such as rice or pasta. Losses are greatest when foods are left out in the light and exposed to the air. Alkaline conditions also increase the destruction of vitamin B$_6$. To minimise losses, make sure foods are fresh and do not overcook.

Deficiency

A deficiency of this vitamin is uncommon except in severe malnutrition where there are deficiencies of all vitamins. If deficiencies of both vitamin B$_6$ and riboflavin occur, the situation is even worse than a lack of either of these vitamins on its own, because riboflavin is involved with the metabolism of B$_6$. Signs of severe deficiency of vitamin B$_6$ include depression, irritability, confusion, and problems of inflammation in the mouth, a swollen red tongue and a line of red denuded skin where the lips close (this problem can also be due to exposure to cold windy weather conditions).

With health problems such as some types of kidney disease, coronary heart disease, alcoholism, breast cancer and diabetes, there is often a decrease in blood levels of pyridoxal 5-phosphate, the most active form of vitamin B_6 within the body. However, in these conditions it is not known whether vitamin B_6 is present in one of its other forms.

Drug interactions

Some prescription drugs can cause a deficiency of vitamin B_6 by forming a complex with pyridoxal 5-phosphate. These drugs include isoniazid (used to treat tuberculosis), cycloserine (used to prevent rejection of transplanted tissue) and penicillamine (used to treat rheumatoid arthritis, some types of kidney stones and heavy metal poisoning). When these drugs are prescribed, a supplement of vitamin B_6 should also be prescribed. Penicillamine sounds like penicillin, but its interactive effects with B_6 do not occur with penicillin antibiotics.

Some anti-convulsant drugs used in epilepsy may also interact with vitamin B_6, with the vitamin reducing the effectiveness of the drug.

Excess

Excess vitamin B_6 can cause damage to nerve endings, leading to a condition known as peripheral neuritis. It is difficult to define the level to be considered excessive. The body needs 2 milligrams a day and doses of 10 milligrams are known to be safe. Very large doses are hazardous but what happens in between is not clear. In one group of women taking B_6, nerve damage developed in seven who took four large doses of between 1000 and 2000 milligrams a day for several months. Other researchers report that daily doses of 500 milligrams over several months may produce peripheral neuropathy. In the United Kingdom, the Committee on Toxicity of Chemicals in Foods, Consumer Products and the Environment recommended that dietary supplements sold over the counter should not have more than 10 milligrams of vitamin B_6. At the time, more than 30 per cent of supplements surveyed had greater levels than this. The new UK recommendations permit pharmacies to sell quantities ranging from 10 to 50 milligrams and anything with greater quantities is only available on a doctor's prescription.

These new regulations have invoked the ire of some sections of the health food and supplement industries. The Council for Responsible Nutrition, a body set up by the supplement industry, conducted a postal survey, sending out more than 10 000 questionnaires asking about vitamin B_6 usage. Of the 1671 replies, most respondents said they took more than 50 milligrams a day and were happy with their supplement. Such a survey is not very comforting to a scientist, especially when harmful effects may develop slowly. Large doses of vitamin B_6 have a drug-like action and should therefore be prescribed on the basis of their safety and proven effectiveness, as with any other drug.

There have been cases where large doses of vitamin B_6 have been used for premenstrual syndrome. The results from placebo-controlled trials have not shown any benefits and there have been some cases of peripheral neuritis as a result of women taking large doses of more than 500 milligrams a day. Without a proven benefit, there is no justification for women to take extra vitamin B_6 for premenstrual syndrome.

Pyridoxine supplements

Some people recommend a supplement of vitamin B_6 for those with high levels of homocysteine in the blood (a known risk factor for coronary heart disease). However, most research indicates that the level of folate, rather than vitamin B_6 is more important to get rid of excess homocysteine. Except in cases of proven deficiency, there is probably no reason for most normally healthy people to take a supplement of vitamin B_6. The reaction of those selling supplements to such statements is to claim that no one is 'normally healthy'. While this can be debated, experts working with this vitamin have stated that the use of vitamin B_6 to treat many of the conditions for which supplement sellers recommend it has not been proven to be beneficial. Since an excess of B_6 can be harmful, it makes sense to check the level present in any supplement to make sure it is not excessive. Almost everyone's needs are covered by a dose of 2 milligrams.

There is an exception to this general statement with alcoholics, up to 30 per cent of whom may have a deficiency of vitamin B_6. Treatment of alcoholism should include supplements of this vitamin, along with other vitamins of the B complex. This should not be extrapolated to mean that anyone who has a few drinks needs vitamin B_6 supplements.

In athletes

For sports people, B_6 supplements are unlikely to be of benefit and may be undesirable. There are a number of studies where vitamin B_6 was given to athletes and the results are somewhat confusing. This is almost certainly due to the fact that exercise itself may alter the blood levels of pyridoxal 5-phosphate, as shown in the high levels apparent immediately after exercise in trained athletes. These return to normal within 30 minutes. The increased levels of the major form of vitamin B_6 in the blood may be due to a release of the vitamin when muscle glycogen is being used for fuel.

The main recommendation that athletes should not take supplements comes from advice from highly respected researchers that supplements of B_6 may cause faster loss of muscle glycogen stores during exercise—a reaction that would be undesirable and could lead to endurance athletes 'hitting the wall' sooner than expected. Supplements of B_6 have also been shown to lower circulating fatty acids during exercise. As these fatty acids are used as fuel, this is another reason not to recommend vitamin B_6 supplements for athletes—at least in quantities larger than the normal recommended dietary intake.

To increase muscle glycogen supplies, athletes should have a diet high in carbohydrate. Those who do not consume enough carbohydrate may break down extra protein for conversion to blood glucose in the process of gluconeogenesis, referred to earlier. If this process is occurring to a large extent, it will increase the amount of vitamin B_6 required, but relying on gluconeogenesis is not a preferred option. It is much better to get glucose from a high-carbohydrate diet than to have a low-carbohydrate diet plus supplementary vitamin B_6. Research shows that a diet high in carbohydrate has many advantages for athletes.

Current research findings

Vitamin B_6 supplements are sometimes recommended

for conditions as diverse as Down's syndrome, autism, premenstrual syndrome, carpal tunnel syndrome and diseases of the nervous system that sometimes accompany long-term diabetes. At this stage, the studies show no conclusive evidence of benefit, but more research is needed.

Pyridoxal 5-phosphate (the active form of B_6 within the body) binds to a particular protein to which human immunodeficiency virus type 1 (HIV–1) also binds. It is therefore possible that vitamin B_6 may have an anti-viral action, at least against some viruses. At this stage, more research is still needed to verify this action and to see if it has clinical significance for those at high risk of HIV–1 infection.

Since pyridoxal 5-phosphate is involved in a great many enzyme reactions within the body, it is unlikely that we fully understand all its roles. Much research is still to be done.

One of the major problems lies in determining a person's vitamin B_6 status. Because the vitamin exists in several forms and is converted into these for specific purposes, you can't just measure the levels of vitamin B_6 in the blood to say whether the person has enough, too much or too little. In general, the level of pyridoxal 5-phosphate in the blood is used as an indicator of B_6 status, but other factors that influence these levels, such as protein intake, smoking and age, must also be considered.

FOLATE OR FOLIC ACID

What it is

Like some other members of the B complex, this vitamin is actually a family of more than 30 compounds. They include folate (proper name is pteroylglutamate), which is the form of the vitamin occurring naturally in foods; folic acid (proper name pteroylglutamic acid), the major form used in supplements and fortified foods; and folacin, a provitamin that is converted to folic acid in the body.

Folic acid was first isolated in 1943 and made in the laboratory in 1945. However, the vitamin was discovered earlier in 1930 by a scientist, Lucy Wills, when she described a factor in yeast that would cure macrocytic anaemia (a type of anaemia where there are very large red blood cells). This unknown factor was first called the 'Wills' factor and was also identified in an extract of liver. The 'Wills' factor was tested in chickens and called vitamin Bc and also in monkeys under the name of vitamin M. By 1941, when the substance was also found in the leaves of spinach, it was called folic acid or folate (from the Latin *folium* meaning 'leaf'). Some scientists also referred to it as vitamin B_{10}, while others dubbed it vitamin B_{11}. When the structure was finally isolated in 1943, the numbers were dropped, although the last vitamin to be identified was later called B_{12}. The numbers that have stuck have been for vitamins B_1, B_2, B_3, B_6 and B_{12}. This has had the unfortunate effect of giving some people the impression that there are only five vitamins in the B complex. Folate, biotin and pantothenic acid are thus forgotten by some.

What it does

Folate has been in the news over the last few years because of its association with conditions such as spina bifida and other birth defects in infants, and also because it plays a role in coronary heart disease, cancer and stroke.

The wide range of folate's involvement is because it has a role in many basic aspects of human biochemistry. These include the production of nucleic acids needed in several steps in synthesising DNA and the formation of a sulphur-containing amino acid called methionine. Folate is also involved in more than 100 biochemical reactions within the body. The synthesis of phospholipids in cell membranes, the growth of cells (including red blood cells) and the removal of certain molecules that can create hazards if they build up to high levels in the body, all involve folate.

Cardiovascular risk

The intimate connections between folate and the sulphur-containing amino acids methionine and homocysteine are the reason for folate's importance in cardiovascular risk.

Homocysteine has been recognised as a risk factor for coronary heart disease since the 1970s, but it was largely ignored until recently because most emphasis was given to cholesterol as the major risk factor. However, many people who have had coronary heart attacks have normal levels of cholesterol. High levels of a risk factor such as homocysteine can help explain some previously unexplained heart attacks and strokes.

Homocysteine is converted within the body into cysteine (another amino acid) and methionine; the latter conversion requiring folate and vitamin B_{12}. Vitamin B_6 is also involved in the metabolism of homocysteine, and all three vitamins (folate, B_6 and B_{12}) are involved in converting homocysteine back to methionine. When blood levels of homocysteine rise, the risk of cardiovascular disease (including coronary heart disease and stroke) increases. More than 20 studies have also shown that when blood levels of folate, B_6 and B_{12} are low, homocysteine levels are undesirably high. Of the three, folate may be the most crucial in controlling undesirably high levels of homocysteine.

A diet high in animal protein foods, such as meat and eggs, will contribute a high load of methionine. Such a diet does not favour those with an impaired ability to convert methionine to homocysteine and then metabolise homocysteine further. The link between homocysteine and methionine also provides an extra reason (in addition to saturated fat) as to why diets high in animal foods can increase the risk of cardiovascular disease in some people, whereas plant foods (with their lower levels of methionine), are protective.

Those with cardiovascular disease have about 30 per cent higher levels of homocysteine in the blood than the rest of the population. After giving such people a dose of methionine, they are twelve times more likely to have an abnormal homocysteine concentration than the average person. Some people, due to their genetic make-up, have trouble clearing methionine and homocysteine from their blood. This could be due to a lack of folate or a genetic defect which means that such people need larger quantities of folate than normal.

Connection with vitamin B_{12}

A number of folate's other roles are also intimately connected with those of vitamin B_{12}, and in cases of B_{12} deficiency, the level of folate within body cells decreases. Both vitamins play a part in many chemical reactions in the body and some nutrition researchers express concern that an excess of folate (from supplements or foods fortified with folate) may mask a deficiency of vitamin B_{12}. Whether this is of practical importance is not yet known, but the potential problem has often been raised as a reason against adding folate to a variety of processed foods.

Many elderly people suffer from a type of anaemia and nerve damage due to a deficiency of vitamin B_{12} because they lack a factor needed for vitamin B_{12} to be absorbed from the small intestine. Often no symptoms are apparent at first and if these people inadvertently take high doses of folate, the anaemia may be cured, but neurological damage from a lack of B_{12} may not be detected until it reaches an advanced stage. This situation may arise if the total folate intake exceeds 1000 micrograms a day.

Neural tube defects

Much of the publicity surrounding folate in recent years has concerned its role in preventing neural tube defects, especially the most common of these, spina bifida. In this condition, one or more bones in the spine don't develop properly, leaving a gap which can allow damage to the spinal cord and nerves.

From the early 1980s, researchers conducting a variety of trials have found that women given folate (generally in doses of 200 to 400 micrograms) in the first six weeks of pregnancy, have a lower incidence of babies with neural tube defects. The timing is important because the neural tube closes by the end of the sixth week after the last period, and many women have not even had their pregnancy confirmed at this stage.

Women who have already had one baby with a neural tube defect are at high risk of having another. Researchers have found that a high dose supplement of 4 milligrams (4000 micrograms) of folate taken daily in the early weeks of pregnancy reduces the chance of having the next infant similarly affected by about 70 per cent. In most cases, women in this situation do not have unusually low blood levels of folate or an especially low intake of folate from food. However, for some as yet unexplained reason, a drug-like dose of the vitamin (20 times the usual recommended dietary intake) overcomes a genetic maternal metabolic defect and increases the chances of protecting the infant against spina bifida. Such high levels of folate are not achievable from foods.

There seems little doubt that spina bifida is due to a genetic abnormality in the way the body uses folate. A poor dietary intake of folate exacerbates this, although it is obviously not the only factor involved. Women who have had an affected pregnancy also have lower blood levels of vitamin B_{12}, a cofactor in the way the body uses folate to deliver the amino acid methionine to the foetus. Some researchers now believe that vitamin B_{12} is more important than folate, but it is more likely that both vitamins are involved.

There are almost certainly some environmental influences on neural tube defects. For example, the incidence is much higher in Australia than in the United States or the United Kingdom. We also know that Mexican women have twice as many pregnancies affected by neural tube defects as other women, but this only occurs when they go through their pregnancy in Mexico. When Mexican women move to the USA, their incidence of neural tube defects decreases. In one study, Mexican women in Mexico who took folic acid supplements had a higher risk of neural tube defects than those not taking the supplements. The number of women taking supplements was small and this study on its own is not enough to undermine the conclusion of most studies that increased folate is an advantage during the early stages of pregnancy, but it does highlight the importance of continuing to look for other factors besides folate.

It is also possible that some other factor may be accompanying the incidence of neural tube defects. Farm pesticides have been suspected since a Norwegian study found that spina bifida was two to three times more common in farming families exposed to pesticides than in non-farming families in the same area.

Recently, a paper published in the *Lancet* medical journal in Britain estimated that for every 1000 women taking folate who became pregnant, there would be ten fewer birth defects but almost twice as many miscarriages as usually occur. Does folate perhaps work in preventing neural tube defects by increasing the number of affected babies that the body aborts? Some researchers don't believe so, citing other studies that have not shown similar findings.

However, there is evidence that women taking folate have a higher rate of multiple births. The reasons for this are unclear. It is possible that women who take folate supplements are better educated and delay having children to a later stage of their lives when multiple births may be more common. Or the fact that they have used oral contraceptives for many years may play a role.

Cancer

Folate is important in the way cells multiply in the body and may also help prevent mutations in genes that can be involved in the early stages of cancer.

Folate also helps cancer cells grow, and an anti-cancer drug called methotrexate is made to be very similar to folate so that it will interfere with the action of folate and prevent the growth of rapidly dividing cancer cells.

The major natural dietary sources of folate are fruits and vegetables. For a while, many researchers assumed that the lower death rates from cancers and cardiovascular disease among those who ate the most fruits and vegetables was due to vitamins C and E and beta carotene in these products. As discussed in the chapters on these vitamins, such assumptions, tragically, were wrong. However, we still do not know if the vital factor in fruits and vegetables could be folate. It is also possible, of course, that the protective effects of fruits and vegetables come from the many hundreds of anti-oxidants they contain.

One of the problems of giving large doses of folate in any prospective cancer prevention program is that the quantity and form of folate that prevents mutations, or helps existing cancer cells to grow, is not clear.

Mood

Studies of psychiatric patients suffering from depression show they have lower levels of folate in the blood than other psychiatric patients. At this stage, it is not known whether folate deficiency produces depression or whether depression leads to lower folate levels, possibly due to poor appetite and poor food selection. Until further research is carried out to establish possible mechanisms, it may be wise to consider folate status in those suffering from depression.

How much you need

The recommended dietary intake of folate is as follows:

Age	RDI (micrograms)
Breast-fed or bottle-fed	50
7–12 months	75
1–7 years	100
Boys and girls, 8–11 years	150
Boys and girls, 12–18 years	200
Men, all ages	200
Women, all ages	200
Pregnancy	400
Lactation	350

There is a major problem in deciding exact needs for folate because there are so many different isomers of the vitamin.

Where it is found

Folate is found in liver and kidney, vegetables, wholegrain cereals, nuts, fruit and legumes. It is also added to many breakfast cereals and some breads.

Food	Folate content (micrograms)
Breads, grains and cereals	
Barley, wholegrain, raw, $\frac{1}{4}$ cup	22
Bran, wheat, 1 tablespoon, 8 g	20
Bread, folate enriched, 1 slice, 30 g	66*
Bread, white, 1 slice, 30 g	9

Food	Folate content (micrograms)
Bread, wholemeal, 1 slice, 30 g	13
Flour, white, 1 cup, 125 g	27
Flour, wholemeal, 1 cup, 130 g	66
Oats, rolled, raw, $\frac{1}{2}$ cup, 50 g	30
Pasta, egg noodles, cooked, 1 cup, 180 g	2
Pasta, white, cooked, 1 cup, 180 g	7
Pasta, wholemeal, cooked, 1 cup, 180 g	13
Rice, brown, cooked, 1 cup, 180 g	18
Rice, white, cooked, 1 cup, 180 g	5
Rye flour, 1 cup, 130 g	101
Soy flour, low-fat, 1 cup, 150 g	615
Wheat germ, 1 tablespoon, 10 g	33
Breakfast cereals	
Allbran, average serve, 45 g	100*
Branflakes, 30 g	100*
Cornflakes, 30 g	100*
Golden wheats, 2, 30 g	100*
Just Right®, average serve, 45 g	100*
Lite Start*®, average serve, 45 g	100*
Mini wheats, all flavours, 30 g	100*
Muesli, Komplete, oven baked, 45 g	100*
Muesli, natural, average serve, 60 g	84
Nutrigrain®, 30 g	50*
Rice Bubbles®, 30 g	50*
Oats, rolled, cooked, average serve, 300 g	20
Sultana Bran®, 45 g	100*
Weetbix, 2 biscuits, 30 g	100*
Dairy products	
Cheese, average of main varieties, 50 g	20
Cheese, cottage, 50 g	13
Cheese, soy, 50 g	18
Cream, average serve, 50 g	3
Cream, sour, 1 tablespoon	3
Fromage frais, fruit-flavoured, 150 g	22

Food	Folate content (micrograms)
Ice cream, 100 mL	5
Milk, cow's, regular or skim, 1 cup	15
Milk, goat's, 1 cup	3
Milk, sheep's, 1 cup	13
Yoghurt, fruit, 200 g	20
Yoghurt, fruit, low-fat, 200 g	38
Yoghurt, natural, regular or low-fat, 200 g	36
Meat, poultry and eggs	
Beef, cooked, average serve, 150 g	22
Chicken, average serve, 150 g	15
Duck, average serve, 150 g	15
Egg, hen, boiled, 1	20
Egg, duck, 1 average	22
Kidney, lamb, cooked, 100 g	80
Lamb, cooked, average serve, 150 g	8
Liver, chicken, cooked, 100 g	500
Liver, lamb, cooked, 100 g	240
Liver, ox, cooked, 100 g	290
Pork, cooked, average serve, 150 g	8
Rabbit, cooked, 150g with bone	3
Sausages, grilled, 2	6
Veal, cooked, average serve, 150 g	6
Fish and seafood	
Crab flesh, cooked, 100 g	20
Fish, average fillet, grilled, 200 g	25
Mussels, fresh, cooked, 10	54
Mussels, green-lipped, 6	80
Oysters, fresh, 6	12
Salmon, grilled, 200 g	38
Salmon, pink or red, canned, 100 g	14
Sardines, canned, 100 g	8
Tuna, canned, 100 g	5
Tuna, fresh, 200 g	30

Food	Folate content (micrograms)
Nuts and seeds	
Almonds, 50 g	24
Brazil nuts, 50 g	10
Cashews, 50 g	34
Coconut, 50 g	13
Hazelnuts, 50 g	36
Macadamias, 50 g	14
Peanut butter, 1 tablespoon	15
Peanuts, raw with skin, 50 g	55
Peanuts, roasted and salted, 50 g	26
Pecans, 50 g	20
Pine nuts, 50 g	27
Pistachios, 50 g	29
Pumpkin seeds, 1 tablespoon	25
Sesame seeds, 2 teaspoons	10
Sunflower seeds, 1 tablespoon	47
Tahini paste, 1 tablespoon	28
Walnuts, 50 g	33
Fruit	
Apple, 1 average	2
Apricots, 2 average	6
Apricots, dried, 6	8
Avocado, $\frac{1}{2}$ medium	11
Banana, 1 average	15
Blackberries and other berries, 100 g	33
Cherries, 200 g	10
Dates, dried, 6	15
Grapefruit, $\frac{1}{2}$ medium	39
Grapes, 200 g	4
Kiwi fruit, 1 average	trace
Mango, 1 average	7
Melon, honeydew, 200 g	118
Melon, rockmelon, 200 g	48
Melon, watermelon, 200 g	6

Food	Folate content (micrograms)
Orange, 1 medium	40
Peach, 1 average	5
Pear, 1 medium	12
Pineapple, 1 slice, 150 g	15
Plums, 2 medium	5
Prunes, 6	5
Raisins, 50 g	5
Sultanas, 50 g	13
Strawberries, $\frac{1}{2}$ punnet, 125 g	25
Vegetables	
Artichoke, globe, 1 medium	36
Asparagus, steamed, 6 spears	66
Beans, broad, fresh, cooked, 100 g	32
Beans, green, cooked, 100 g	57
Bean sprouts, mung, raw, 1 cup	56
Beetroot, cooked, $\frac{1}{2}$ cup	135
Broccoli, cooked, average serve, 100 g	64
Brussels sprouts, cooked, 6	99
Cabbage, green, cooked, 1 cup	39
Cabbage, green, raw, 1 cup	67
Cabbage, red, cooked, 1 cup	40
Capsicum, green, raw, 100 g	36
Capsicum, red, raw, 100 g	21
Carrot, mature, cooked, 1 medium	20
Celeriac, cooked, $\frac{1}{2}$ cup	30
Cauliflower, cooked, 1 cup	60
Endive, raw, average serve, 40 g	56
Kale, cooked, 1 cup	77
Leek, cooked, $\frac{1}{2}$ cup	30
Lettuce, 4 leaves	50
Mushrooms, fried, 100 g	11
Mushrooms, raw, 100 g	44
Okra, fried, 75 g	61
Onion, cooked, 1 medium	30

Food	Folate content (micrograms)
Parsley, $\frac{1}{2}$ cup	40
Parsnip, cooked, 1 medium	50
Peas, sugar snap or snow, 1 cup	10
Peas, green, frozen, cooked, 100 g	47
Potato, 1 average, cooked, 180 g	40
Pumpkin, average serve, 120 g	12
Silverbeet, cooked, $\frac{1}{2}$ cup	90
Spinach, English, cooked, 100 g	90
Spinach, English, raw, 100g	150
Sweet corn kernels, 100 g	40
Tomato, raw, 1 medium, 150 g	25
Tomato puree, $\frac{1}{2}$ cup	68
Watercress, raw, 1 cup	35
Zucchini, cooked, 1 medium	20

Legumes

Food	Folate content (micrograms)
Beans, black eye, cooked, 1 cup	330
Beans, kidney, canned, 1 cup	12
Beans, kidney, cooked, 1 cup	67
Chickpeas, cooked, 1 cup	96
Lentils, cooked, 1 cup	50
Pinto beans, cooked, 1 cup	245
Soy beans, cooked, 1 cup	96

Take-away foods

Food	Folate content (micrograms)
Barbecued chicken, $\frac{1}{4}$	10
Bean salad, $\frac{1}{2}$ cup	50
Beer, bitter, 250 mL	8
Beer, lager, 250 mL	30
Chips, hot, average serve, 150 g	28
Coleslaw, $\frac{1}{2}$ cup	34
Fish, battered and fried, 1 piece, 150 g	8
Hamburger, 1	28
Hamburger, fast food chain, 1	14
Hamburger with cheese, 1	31
Hamburger with egg, 1	65

Food	Folate content (micrograms)
Meat pie, 1	9
Peanut brittle, 50 g	18
Pizza, $\frac{1}{2}$ medium, average, 300 g	100
Potato crisps, 50 g	19
Potato salad, $\frac{1}{2}$ cup	30
Sausage roll, 1	6
Miscellaneous	
Apple juice, 250 mL	10
Chocolate, 50 g	6
Fish sauce, 1 tablespoon	10
Marmite, 1 teaspoon	100*
Orange juice, 250 mL	50
Pasta sauce (tomato-based), $\frac{3}{4}$ cup	18
Soy beverage, 1 cup	48
Tempeh, 50 g	26–38
Tofu, 100 g	15–33
Vegemite, 1 teaspoon	20*
Yeast, dried, 2 teaspoons	400

* Added folate
® Registered trade mark Kellogg (Aust) Pty Ltd
*® Registered trade mark Uncle Toby's

It is not easy to measure the level of folate in foods because the vitamin exists in complex structures. Isolating the different forms of folate from proteins, carbohydrates and dietary fibre is technically difficult and the separation methods can easily destroy the vitamin. The levels of folate in food sometimes differ because of the method of analysis used.

Bioavailability

Certain foods, including breakfast cereals and bread that are fortified with added folate use the monoglutamyl form of folate. Some researchers believe this is more easily absorbed into the body than the polyglutamyl form present naturally in foods. However, this does not negate the importance of natural foods such as fruits and vegetables as sources of folate. One study reported that women taking folic acid supplements or using foods fortified with folic acid had higher levels of folate in their red blood cells than those using fruits and vegetables as natural sources of folate. However, in this study the lower levels of folate in red blood cells in the group using natural food sources of folate could have been due to the simple fact that compliance was poor. Most of the women did not consume the amount of fruits and vegetables suggested! Some have taken this study to mean that folate added to foods is preferable, but it may be even more important to find ways to encourage women to eat more fruits and vegetables.

Factors that can influence the bioavailability of folate include low acid secretion in the stomach, ageing, alcohol, anti-convulsant drugs, non-steroidal inflammatory drugs (often called NSAIDs) and HIV infection. There are also some individual genetic effects that influence how much folate is absorbed from the intestine and also how it is used within the body. These may be important reasons why some women have babies with neural tube defects even though their intake of folate is not significantly different from other women.

There are also other unknown factors in foods that influence how much of their folate is absorbed. For example, some studies from the 1970s found that only 25 to 50 per cent of folate was absorbed from lettuce, oranges, eggs and wheat germ, whereas almost all the folate was absorbed from liver, Lima beans, brewer's yeast and bananas. However, the method of analysing absorption at this time was possibly less accurate than is now possible.

Fortification

In their efforts to reduce neural tube defects, governments in some countries, including Australia, the United States and the United Kingdom, have recommended that some basic foods such as breads, flour and cereals should be fortified with folate. The upper level for folate fortification in Australia has been set at 100 micrograms per serve of a food, half the RDI for the vitamin. This limit on added folate is designed to avoid an intake greater than 1000 micrograms a day in elderly people in whom higher quantities may mask vitamin B_{12} deficiency.

Effect of cooking

Folate is destroyed by heat and oxidation at cooking temperatures greater than 100°C. In vegetables, the presence of vitamin C helps prevent some losses but even so, raw vegetables are always a better source of folate than those that have been cooked. The more water used in cooking vegetables, the greater the losses.

Freezing retains about three-quarters of the folate, although there can be later losses when frozen vegetables are cooked. Steaming results in less loss of the vitamin than boiling. When cooking rice and pasta, losses are also high.

When wheat is ground to white flour, more than 50 per cent of the folate is lost. Folate is currently being added to many breakfast cereals and a few breads. It appears to be fairly stable in these foods, with losses in cereals reported at about 33 to over 50 per cent after twelve months storage, but lower losses over shorter storage times.

Deficiency

It is difficult to define folate deficiency because testing blood serum levels of folate is not always relevant and does not always reveal a true picture of folate status. In most studies, red blood cell folate levels are measured. A number of other tests are also used to measure levels of compounds that require folate for their normal functioning.

A lack of folate is the most likely vitamin deficiency in countries such as Australia. It can occur due to poor dietary intake, alcoholism or poor absorption of the vitamin (which may be a secondary characteristic of some other disease). Folate deficiency may also be more common during pregnancy when rapid cell growth increases requirements.

A full-blown deficiency results in macrocytic or megaloblastic anaemia, which can be detected from a blood sample or by examining bone marrow. In suspected cases, it is also important to test for vitamin B_{12} deficiency, as the symptoms are similar. Macrocytic anaemia is characterised by abnormally large red blood cells.

As discussed earlier, a lack of folate can lead to increased levels of homocysteine in the blood and an increased risk of coronary heart disease and stroke.

There also seems to be a strong connection between folate deficiency and cancer of the lining of the cervix and also with colorectal cancer. In the large Nurses Health Study in Boston, those who had the lowest intake of folate had about three times the incidence of bowel cancer as those with the highest intakes. When this study was done, folate came principally from natural food sources (mostly fruits and vegetables) rather than fortified foods. Studies in animals confirm these findings by showing that colon cancer can be induced faster and with more serious effects when the animals are deficient in folate.

The links between folate deficiency and certain types of cancer almost certainly involve DNA. Folate-deficient cells stop making DNA and are left at a stage of maximal sensitivity to cancer-causing substances in the environment. The cells also fail to repair any damage, and their DNA becomes susceptible to gamma irradiation. Experts think that low levels of folate are related to the initiation stages of cancer, but probably have no effect on the progression of cancer. In other words, once someone has cancer it seems unlikely that taking large doses of folate will be helpful.

Several studies have shown low to deficient red blood cell folate levels in one-sixth to one-third of people suffering from depression. The folate levels were not low enough to show any anaemia. In general, people with low folate levels in red blood cells have more depression than those with normal red blood cell folate level. However, before advising anyone with depression to take folic acid, we should note that studies in both humans and animals have suggested that high doses of folic acid can also increase symptoms such as irritability and malaise. At this stage, no one knows whether folate deficiency produces depression, or whether depression increases losses of folate, so it would be foolish for such people to take folic acid supplements until more is known.

Drug interactions

Long-term use of some anti-convulsants or anti-epileptic drugs such as phenytoin, diphenylhydatoin, phenobarbitone and primidone may lead to a deficiency of folate. When these drugs must be used over long periods, a supplement of folate is advisable. However, the folate supplement may reduce their effects.

Sulfasalazine, used for chronic conditions such as inflammatory bowel disease and rheumatoid arthritis, may also interfere with the way the body absorbs and uses folate. The anti-malarial drug pyrimethamine, the antibiotic trimethoprim (used for treating some urinary tract infections) and some sedatives can also deplete folate levels. Prescription of any of these drugs means that a folate supplement should also be taken.

Excess

Folate seems to be fairly non-toxic. The main adverse effect is a masking of vitamin B_{12} deficiency, as discussed earlier. There were also reports in the 1970s of epileptic symptoms becoming worse when large doses of 15 milligrams a day (more than 70 times the RDI) were used to treat megaloblastic anaemia in people with epilepsy.

Folate supplements

There is probably more evidence to support taking folate supplements than for any other vitamin. The debate is continuing over whether all women of child-bearing age should take folate supplements, or whether more foods should be fortified with folate to increase overall consumption throughout the community.

There is no doubt that the major effects of folate on

the neural tube of an infant occur very early in the pregnancy. It is also a fact that many pregnancies are unplanned, and even when they are planned, we have no way of knowing which women are at a high risk of having an infant with a neural tube defect. For these valid reasons, many doctors advise all women of child-bearing age to take folate supplements. Arguments opposing this look at the fact that foods rich in folate are also excellent sources of other important nutrients that are especially important during pregnancy. If women decide, for example, that they can use folate fortified foods instead of eating vegetables and fruits, their total diet will not be improved.

For women who have had an infant with a neural tube defect, a daily folate supplement containing 400 milligrams is recommended. This is 2000 times the normal recommended dietary intake.

For women who may become pregnant, the recommendations for folate intake of 400 micrograms a day is achievable from a well-chosen diet. Health practitioners who prefer to prescribe a supplement often recommend 500 micrograms (or 0.5 milligrams) because this is the common level in folate supplements. Many multivitamins have insignificant quantities of folate and are not a valid recommendation for their folate content.

Several recent studies have indicated that high levels of folate are not necessary to prevent neural tube defects. One study in the *Lancet* in the United Kingdom, reported that 200 micrograms, or even 100 micrograms could produce important reductions in neural tube defects. Another suggested that only 15 per cent of the population need extra folic acid because they have a genetic defect in producing the enzymes that metabolise folate.

Some gynaecologists advise women who have had a spontaneous abortion, or a history of miscarriages or other problems that end a pregnancy, to delay another pregnancy until they are taking 5 milligrams of folate a day. Such women also need their vitamin B_{12} status checked, in case the high dose of folate masks a deficiency in this vitamin. However, this is unlikely in women of child-bearing age, with the exception of vegans or vegetarians who eat poorly.

For those with high levels of homocysteine

In pharmacological doses, folate decreases homocysteine levels in those with normal or raised levels. Whether this artificial lowering of homocysteine levels is beneficial is not yet known. One study in Northern Ireland added folic acid supplements of 100, 200 and 400 micrograms to the daily diet which already contained an average level of 280 micrograms. Of the three folic acid doses, 200 micrograms reduced homocysteine levels to a greater extent than 100 micrograms, but there was no further increase with the 400 microgram supplement. This useful total daily intake from food plus the supplement was 480 micrograms, a level which could be achieved by a wise choice of healthy foods. Other studies have also shown that consuming more than 400 micrograms of folate results in lower homocysteine levels.

Supplements of folate (6400 micrograms) with or without 20 micrograms cobalamin (B_{12}) given to adults (aged 52 to 82) with osteoarthritis had advantages over nonsteroidal anti-inflammatory drugs (NSAIDs), in increased grip strength with the supplement of both vitamins (folate on its own was not effective) and fewer tender hand joints. There were no side effects with the vitamins but many with NSAIDs.

Current research findings

Research is continuing into the effects of folate on neural tube defects, cardiovascular disease and cancer.

Researchers are also trying to determine the exact dose of folate required to reduce homocysteine levels. A recent trial which used supplements with either 127, 499 or 665 micrograms of folic acid found that the lowest level had no significant effect on plasma homocysteine levels, but either of the two higher levels produced a favourable decrease.

There is also some research looking at a possible role for milk in helping prevent spina bifida. Milk contains a protein that binds to folate, making it easier for the body to absorb the vitamin. Researchers are trying to isolate that protein so it can be combined with added folate to increase the amount absorbed.

CYANOCOBALAMIN OR VITAMIN B$_{12}$

What it is

Vitamin B$_{12}$ is unusual in at least two ways. First, it is not found in plants and secondly, a deficiency is more likely to be due to a failure to absorb the vitamin than to a dietary deficiency, although the latter can certainly occur.

The history of this vitamin is relatively recent. Pernicious anaemia, the disease that occurs with a deficiency of vitamin B$_{12}$, was first described in 1824, but it was 100 years later that a cure was found. In 1926, medical scientists found that the fatal condition could be cured by beef mixed with gastric juice. Large quantities of liver were also used with limited success in treating pernicious anaemia, but beef on its own was ineffective.

The vitamin was finally isolated in 1948, and its chemical structure was fully worked out by Dr Dorothy Hodgkin in 1964, earning her a Nobel Prize in Chemistry.

Vitamin B_{12} is made by micro-organisms and is a group of compounds called corrinoids. Some of these are used by micro-organisms within the human intestine but are not actually useful for humans. The molecule most people refer to as vitamin B_{12} is also known as cyanocobalamin. As this term suggests, it contains the element cobalt (which makes up about 4 per cent of the molecule by weight), and its full name is alpha-(5,6-dimethylbenzimidazolyl)-cobamide cyanide. The three major forms of vitamin B_{12} are 5'-deoxyadenosylcobalamin, hydroxycobalamin and methylcobalamin. They are all soluble in water.

What it does

Vitamin B_{12} is needed, along with folate, by all body cells that make DNA. When B_{12} is lacking the body cannot use folate, so the two vitamins are inextricably linked and both are vital in any times of growth, including repair of all body tissues.

Vitamin B_{12} is especially important for making red blood cells. A lack of B_{12} can be seen in bone marrow cells which become abnormally large (called megaloblasts), although they carry a normal amount of haemoglobin. Their abnormality is due to limited production of DNA and is also related to a lack of folate.

Vitamin B_{12} plays a part in the production of myelin, the sheath that surrounds nerve fibres. This role does not require folate.

One form of B_{12}, hydroxycobalamin, can help detoxify cyanide, a component of cigarette smoke. It is therefore possible that this vitamin may be needed in larger quantities by smokers or those forced to endure passive smoking.

How much you need

Only minute quantities of vitamin B_{12} are needed. One-tenth of a microgram a day may be enough to prevent signs of deficiency, providing there is no impediment to efficient absorption. However, larger quantities are recommended because of inefficiencies in absorption and also to allow for storage. Body stores tend to rise throughout life and this may help provide adequate quantities if absorption decreases later in life.

The recommended dietary intake of vitamin B_{12} is as follows:

Age	RDI (micrograms)
Breast-fed or bottle-fed	0.3
7–12 months	0.7
1–3 years	1.0
4–7 years	1.5
Boys and girls, 8–11 years	1.5
Boys and girls, 12–18 years	2.0
Men, all ages	2.0
Women, all ages	2.0
Pregnancy	3.0
Lactation	2.5

Where it is found

Vitamin B_{12} is the only one of the vitamins, apart from vitamin A, that is not found in plant foods. And unlike vitamin A, which can be made in the body from beta carotene in plant foods, vitamin B_{12} must be supplied ready made. Although some vegans maintain that the vitamin can be made by bacteria in the human intestine, this is doubtful and it is unlikely that enough could ever be supplied from intestinal bacteria. However, some B_{12} may be obtained from dirt and from foods and hands contaminated with micro-organisms coming from faecal materials. These sources are obviously not recommended, although they may have sustained people against B_{12} deficiency in some situations. Fermented foods such as tempeh, and some types of seaweed may contain some vitamin B_{12}. Some vitamin B_{12} is also excreted from the body in bile and this may be re-absorbed in the large intestine.

Vitamin B_{12} exists in many forms, including some that are not available to the body. For example, the B_{12} in spirulina and also in the herb comfrey cannot be absorbed and used by humans. These unavailable forms of vitamin B_{12} are known as B_{12} analogues and are useless. Studies are continuing into the B_{12} content of mushrooms to see how much of the vitamin that migrates from the compost in which the mushrooms are grown is in a form that can be absorbed by the body. Research to date shows that the amount of vitamin B_{12} in mushrooms would fall far short of the recommended dietary intake of the vitamin.

The best sources of vitamin B_{12} are organ meats such as liver and kidney, clams, oysters and other seafood and egg yolks. Meats and milk contain moderate amounts. Tempeh (made from fermented soy beans) and soy beverages and soy yoghurts fortified with vitamin B_{12} are sources for vegetarians, but pregnant women who eat no animal products should take a B_{12} supplement.

Food	Vitamin B_{12} content (micrograms)
Breads, grains and cereals	
All types	0
Dairy products	
Cheese, average of main varieties, 50 g	0.80
Cheese, cottage, 50 g	0.35
Cheese, ricotta, 50 g	0.15
Cheese, soy, 50 g	1.25
Cream, regular or sour, 50 g	0.10
Fromage frais, fruit flavoured, 150 g	0.25
Ice cream, 100 mL	0.25
Milk, cow's, regular or skim, 1 cup	1.00
Milk, goat's, 1 cup	0.25
Milk, sheep's, 1 cup	1.50
Yoghurt, fruit, 200 g	0.20
Yoghurt, natural, 200 g	0.40
Meat, poultry and eggs	
Beef, cooked, average serve, 150g	3
Chicken, average serve, 150 g	trace
Duck, average serve, 150 g	4.5
Egg, hen, boiled, 1	0.60
Egg, duck, 1 average	2.8
Kidney, lamb, cooked, 100 g	79.0
Lamb, cooked, average serve, 150 g	3.0
Liver, chicken, cooked, 100 g	49.0
Liver, lamb, cooked, 100 g	81.0
Liver, ox, cooked, 100 g	110.0
Pork, cooked, average serve, 150 g	3.0
Rabbit, cooked, average serve, 150 g	9.0
Sausages, grilled, 2	1.5

Food	Vitamin B$_{12}$ content (micrograms)
Veal, cooked, average serve, 150 g	1.5
Fish and seafood	
Fish, average fillet, grilled, 200 g	2.0
Mussels, fresh, cooked, 10	33.0
Mussels, green-lipped, 6, 150 g	46.0
Oysters, fresh, 6	18.0
Pipi, fresh, raw, 6	18.0
Salmon, grilled, 200 g	10.0
Salmon, pink or red, canned, 100 g	4.0
Sardines, canned, 100 g	28.0
Tuna, canned, 100 g	5.0
Tuna, fresh, 200 g	8.0
Nuts and seeds	
Any type	0
Fruit	
Any type	0
Vegetables	
Any type	0
Legumes	
Any type	0
Take-away foods	
Barbecued chicken, $\frac{1}{4}$	0.8
Fish, battered and fried, 1 piece, 150 g	1.6
Hamburger, 1	1.3
Hamburger, fast food chain, average, 1	2.8
Hamburger with cheese, 1	1.8
Hamburger with egg, 1	1.9
Pizza, $\frac{1}{2}$ medium, average, 300 g	1.4
Miscellaneous	
Fish sauce, 1 tablespoon	0.1

Food	Vitamin B$_{12}$ content (micrograms)
Marmite, 1 teaspoon	0.5
So Good smoothie, 250 mL	1.0
Soy beverage, unfortified, 1 cup	0
Soy beverage, fortified, 1 cup	1.0
Tempeh, 50 g	0.5
Tofu, 100 g	0
UP and GO breakfast drink, 250 mL	0.5
Vegetarian meals, fortified (check label), per serve	0.6–1.0

Absorption

The absorption of vitamin B$_{12}$ from food is somewhat complicated. In the stomach, acid and an enzyme called pepsin free the B$_{12}$ from food. The vitamin then attaches itself to swallowed salivary protein and cells in the stomach release a glycoprotein called intrinsic factor. When the stomach contents pass to the small intestine, the intrinsic factor allows the vitamin B$_{12}$ to be absorbed from the ileum (the last part of the small intestine). To complicate matters, the pancreas must also be functioning normally to produce the enzyme trypsin which can digest the salivary protein and free the vitamin B$_{12}$ for absorption. This last step can only occur in the strongly alkaline environment of the small intestine. Free calcium ions are also needed for vitamin B$_{12}$ to be absorbed. In some diseases of the pancreas, vitamin B$_{12}$ cannot be absorbed, although the problem can be partially overcome by giving pancreatic extract, calcium and bicarbonate.

Effect of cooking

Vitamin B$_{12}$ is fairly stable to light, oxygen, heat and acidic conditions and these factors cause little loss of the vitamin. There is some loss if foods are cooked in alkaline conditions. In some parts of the world, meat is softened by sprinkling with bicarbonate of soda, an alkaline substance that destroys several vitamins, including some vitamin B_{12}.

When milk is pasteurised, less than 10 per cent of the vitamin B_{12} is lost. Greater losses occur if milk is boiled, especially if it is boiled for long periods as occurs in making some Indian desserts.

Deficiency

The liver stores about 1000 times the estimated daily needs for vitamin B_{12} and some is recycled each day within the body. For this reason, signs of deficiency develop slowly and it may be many years before any symptoms appear. Unfortunately, this can mean the problem may be ignored.

A deficiency of vitamin B_{12} eventually leads to macrocytic (or megaloblastic) anaemia, although this can also be due to a deficiency of folate. Because of its destructive nature, the anaemia has often been referred to as 'pernicious' anaemia.

Signs of neurological damage are not apparent early in the condition. Later there is some tingling or sense of vibration. The gait becomes unsteady, the person lacks a sense of their position and begins to walk with an unsteady step. Those who are deficient are also likely to be irritable and to miss some detail from the central area of their visual field. Later signs include emotional instability, feeling sleepy and confused.

In the absence of sufficient vitamin B_{12}, when branched-chain amino acids are not metabolised properly and begin to appear in the nervous system, one called methylmalonic acid is excreted in the urine. Measuring the levels of this substance can be used to define vitamin B_{12} deficiency. A deficiency can also be diagnosed by measuring levels of the circulating proteins in the blood serum that deliver vitamin B_{12} to all cells that synthesise DNA. The level of these particular proteins is low before damage has occurred in brain and nerve cells, so testing them in vegetarians and other susceptible people, including the very elderly, might be a wise move.

Another test involves giving radioactive vitamin B_{12} and measuring how much is absorbed. This is known as the Schillings test.

Measuring total blood levels of vitamin B_{12} is not useful in the early stages of a deficiency because most B_{12} is bound to a protein that does not show up in the usual tests.

Vegetarians

A deficiency of vitamin B_{12} can easily occur in vegans, who consume no animal products. During pregnancy, B_{12} needs are high and sufficient supplies are crucial for the development of the baby's nervous system and also for the mother. Women who do eat animal products should take a vitamin B_{12} supplement, especially during pregnancy.

Some recent studies in vegetarians who consume dairy products and eggs, but no meat, found levels of vitamin B_{12} were also lower than desirable. Soy beverages with added B_{12}, as well as more yoghurt, milk and eggs can help, but some vegetarians may need a supplement, especially during pregnancy and lactation.

Babies born to vegan mothers can easily lack vitamin B_{12}, mainly because levels in the mother's milk reflect her own low levels.

Much of the concern about vitamin B_{12} in vegans and vegetarians is because their diets are usually so high in folate that the symptoms of anaemia are not apparent. However, damage to the body's nerves continues silently until symptoms become obvious when the deficiency is advanced.

Intrinsic factor

In examining the action of vitamin B_{12}, we must consider 'intrinsic factor', the substance that is essential for B_{12} to be absorbed from the ileum (part of the small intestine). Without intrinsic factor, vitamin B_{12} given by mouth is not absorbed, although if very large doses are given, a very small percentage may passively diffuse across the intestine.

A lack of intrinsic factor is probably due to an auto-immune reaction that can destroy the glands in the stomach that produce it. No one understands why this occurs, but it becomes more common as people age and many elderly people produce very little intrinsic factor. As a result, they can develop pernicious anaemia.

Many older people who have low levels of B_{12} in their blood seem to produce ample quantities of intrinsic factor. Their deficiency occurs because the stomach does not produce enough acid and pepsin which are needed to free B_{12} from foods.

Vitamin B_{12} deficiency may also occur if the stomach or ileum are removed in surgery. In such cases, the vitamin must be given by injection.

Drugs

Drugs such as slow-release potassium, cochicine (used to treat inflammation in joints, including gout) and biguanides (used in some types of diabetes) may interfere with the absorption of B_{12}. If these drugs cannot be avoided and are taken long-term, an occasional vitamin B_{12} injection may be required.

One of the oral diabetic tablets, metformin, causes malabsorption of B_{12}, although this can be overcome by giving milk or calcium carbonate tablets.

Excess

Doses of vitamin B_{12} more than 1000 times the RDI do not seem to cause any problems. The low toxicity may reflect the fact that the vitamin is present only in minute quantities in the body.

However, large doses of vitamin C (more than 500 milligrams) may have an adverse effect on the absorption of vitamin B_{12}, and people who take such high doses of vitamin C may develop a vitamin B_{12} deficiency. The problem is not resolved by also taking B_{12} supplements, because high quantities of vitamin C convert B_{12} to analogues with an anti-vitamin B_{12} action. In the presence of iron, vitamin C is a potent pro-oxidant, generating production of large quantities of free radicals, some of which damage vitamin B_{12} and also destroy the intrinsic factor needed for its absorption. Much of the work in this area has been done by Dr Victor Herbert, one of the world's leading experts on vitamin B_{12}.

Vitamin B_{12} supplements

There seems to be no justification for supplements or injections of vitamin B_{12} in people who consume animal products, unless there is a proven deficiency. However, vegans, people who eat no animal products at all, are likely to become deficient in vitamin B_{12}, and a supplement is a good idea, especially for pregnant women and children.

Vegetarians

Even among vegetarians who consume yoghurt, eggs or milk, there is a significant number who are deficient in vitamin B_{12} and should take a supplement. This is especially important for women during pregnancy and lactation. Children who are not given animal products should be given soy beverage fortified with vitamin B_{12}, or a B_{12} supplement.

Some soy products and cereals are fortified with vitamin B_{12} and, providing vegetarians consume these products, an extra supplement may not be necessary.

Elderly people

Some researchers believe that blood levels of B_{12} are related to dementia and Alzheimer's disease in the elderly. A recent five-year longitudinal study of people aged 75 to 85 found no such relationship and reported that those with lower blood serum levels of B_{12} had a lower incidence of both Alzheimer's disease and dementia than those with higher B_{12} levels.

For elderly people, a supplement of vitamin B_{12} taken by mouth is not usually useful because poor absorption is generally the major problem. When levels are low, whether deficiency occurs because of a lack of intrinsic factor or poor absorption due to a lack of acid and pepsin, injections of vitamin B_{12} are needed. Where some absorption is still occurring, as is usually the case, an injection of 100 micrograms once a month is advisable.

When megaloblastic anaemia is present, a larger dose of 1000 micrograms twice a week is needed, until the blood tests show normal levels. This is followed by an injection every six weeks to maintain levels.

There is some evidence that adding a B_{12} supplement to a folate supplement may help reduce high levels of homocysteine in the blood. This would then be expected to reduce the incidence of cardiovascular disease. The dose of B_{12} required appears to be 0.5 to 1.0 milligrams, taken with 500 micrograms of folate. These quantities could easily be obtained from the diet.

If cyanide poisoning inadvertently occurs, a large injection of hydrocobalamin can help to soak up the toxic material and increase the chances of survival.

In athletes

Vitamin B_{12} given by injection is common in some sports people, although there is little justification for using it. One sports medicine doctor I knew maintained that the weekly jab was psychologically good for his football team, although he could never explain why. Body builders commonly take the vitamin orally, believing it will help build muscle (it won't). Some endurance athletes also think that because vitamin B_{12} has a role in red blood cells, it will be an advantage during long stressful events. However, in spite of widespread use, there is no data that vitamin B_{12} helps athletic performance and no study has yet shown a difference in performance between athletes given B_{12} and those given a placebo.

Current research findings

Researchers are still trying to untangle the way vitamin B_{12} works with folate. Although many of the mechanisms are understood, there is still some fine biochemical tuning to be done, especially in developing better methods to detect the early stages of B_{12} deficiency.

There is also research into vitamin B_{12} and AIDS. About half of those who have AIDS have low levels of vitamin B_{12} with some changes in red blood cells that can be reversed by giving extra B_{12}.

BIOTIN

What it is

Probably the least known member of the B complex, biotin was first synthesised in the vitamin heydays of the 1940s. There are eight different forms of the vitamin, but only one, known as d-(+)-biotin, is useful for humans. It is usually referred to as D-biotin. The molecule itself is complicated, but its shape is responsible for the way a deficiency usually occurs (see below). As biotin is widely distributed in both animal and plant foods, and the quantities required are minute, almost everyone who has food to eat gets enough of it. Biotin is also made by bacteria living in the intestine, and this may be the major source for most people.

Biotin has hit the limelight a few times when a deficiency has occurred in someone with great enthusiasm for raw eggs. Egg white contains a substance called avidin which attaches with amazing tenacity to the particular shape of the biotin molecule, making the vitamin unavailable. If egg white is cooked, the avidin is denatured and the biotin is freed. With the exception of devotees of raw eggs, biotin deficiency rarely occurs and this probably accounts for many people being unaware of its existence.

What it does

Biotin is needed as a co-enzyme in many biochemical systems within the body. These include the body's ability to use dissolved carbon dioxide in a series of reactions involved in making fatty acids and also converting protein into glucose.

How much you need

A recommended dietary intake of biotin has not been set, mainly because no one yet knows how much is needed. The values given below represent a safe and adequate intake as described by the National Research Council in the United States.

Age	Safe and adequate intake (micrograms)
Pre-term infants	5
Infants, under 6 months	10
Infants, 6–12 months	15
Children, 1–3 years	20
Children, 4–6 years	25
Children, 7–10 years	30
Boys and girls, over 11 years	30–100
Adults, all ages	30–100

Because biotin is also made by bacteria in the intestine, the true requirements from the diet may be less than these figures. The bacterial source of biotin has often been ignored because it is variable and relatively unstudied. During tube feeding, especially if antibiotics which kill off intestinal bacteria are being used, bacterial synthesis may not occur. This could also influence the absorption of biotin. By contrast, if the bacterial mass is increased by particular diets, bacteria may contribute significant quantities of biotin.

If biotin is unavailable to the body because it is bound to avidin, requirements might be higher.

Biotin is concentrated in breast milk, but without enough data, no extra amount has been recommended during lactation. However, it would seem wise for breast-feeding women to avoid eating large quantities of raw egg white. The vitamin also crosses the placenta, although it seems to accumulate in the placenta and only small amounts are detectable in the baby before birth. No extra amount is recommended during pregnancy.

Where it is found

Animals do not produce biotin themselves but either get it directly from what they eat or from bacteria, yeasts, moulds and algae. Like humans, their biotin is often obtained from bacteria living in the intestine.

Many foods have not been analysed for their biotin content, but the best sources include liver, nuts, peanuts and eggs. Vegetables are sometimes said to be a good source, but figures are not available for many varieties. Grains and cereal products, dairy products, meat and fish contain only small quantities.

Food	Biotin content (micrograms)
Breads, grains and cereals	
Bran, wheat, 1 tablespoon, 8 g	4

Food	Biotin content (micrograms)
Bread, wholemeal, 1 slice, 30 g	2
Flour, white, 1 cup, 125 g	1
Flour, wholemeal, 1 cup, 130 g	9
Oats, rolled, raw, $\frac{1}{2}$ cup, 50 g	10
Rice, white, cooked, 1 cup, 180 g	2
Rye flour, 1 cup, 130 g	8
Wheat germ, 1 tablespoon, 10 g	3
Breakfast cereals	
Allbran, $\frac{1}{2}$ cup, 40 g	10*
Branflakes, average serve, 45 g	5*
Cornflakes, average serve, 40 g	2*
Muesli, natural, average serve, 60 g	9*
Oats, rolled, cooked, average serve, 300 g	6*
Weetbix, 2 biscuits, 30 g	2*.
Dairy products	
Cheese, average of main varieties, 50 g	2
Cream, regular or sour, 50 g	1
Custard, egg, $\frac{1}{2}$ cup	8
Ice cream, 100 mL	2
Milk, cow's, regular or skim, 1 cup	5
Milk, goat's, 1 cup	8
Milk, human, 100 mL	1
Milk, sheep's, 1 cup	6
Yoghurt, fruit, regular or low-fat, 200 g	4
Yoghurt, natural, regular or low-fat, 200 g	6
Meat, poultry and eggs	
Bacon, grilled, 2 rashers, 60 g	1
Beef or veal, cooked, average serve, 150 g	trace
Chicken or duck, average serve, 150 g	6
Egg, hen, 1	15
Kidney, lamb, cooked, 100 g	42
Lamb, cooked, average serve, 150 g	3
Liver, chicken, cooked, 100 g	170

* values for UK products

Food	Biotin content (micrograms)
Liver, lamb, cooked, 100 g	41
Liver, ox, cooked, 100 g	50
Pork, cooked, average serve, 150 g	5
Sausages, 2 grilled	3
Fish and seafood	
Crab flesh, cooked, 100 g	7
Fish, average fillet, grilled, 200 g	3
Mussels, fresh, cooked, 10	13
Oysters, fresh, 6	9
Salmon, grilled, 200 g	18
Salmon, pink or red, canned, 100 g	9
Sardines, canned, 100 g	1
Tuna, canned, 100 g	3
Nuts and seeds	
Almonds, 50 g	32
Brazil nuts, 50 g	6
Cashews, 50 g	6
Chestnuts, 50 g	1
Hazelnuts, 50 g	38
Macadamias, 50 g	3
Peanut butter, 1 tablespoon	27
Peanuts, raw with skin, 50 g	36
Peanuts, roasted and salted, 50 g	51
Sesame seeds, 2 teaspoons	1
Tahini paste, 1 tablespoon	3
Walnuts, 50 g	10
Fruit	
Average piece, fresh	1
Avocado, $\frac{1}{2}$ medium	4
Berries, $\frac{1}{2}$ punnet	3
Orange juice, 1 cup	3
Vegetables	
Average serve of most vegetables	1

Food	Biotin content (micrograms)
Artichoke, globe, 100 g	4
Mushrooms, 100 g	12
Peas, edible pods, cooked, 100 g	4
Tomato puree, $\frac{1}{2}$ cup	8
Legumes	
Beans, baked, canned, 1 cup	5
Beans, black eye, cooked, 1 cup	14
Beans, kidney, canned, 1 cup	1
Soy beans, cooked, 1 cup	40
Tempeh, 50 g	27
Miscellaneous	
Chocolate, 50 g	2
Peanut brittle, 50 g	12
Yeast, dried, 2 teaspoons	20

Effect of cooking

Biotin is stable to heat and is retained even when foods such as eggs are dried to make egg powder.

Deficiency

The most commonly reported cases of biotin deficiency have occurred in people who have consumed large quantities of raw egg white. Concerned about the fat and cholesterol in egg yolk, and keen to increase their protein intake, some body builders add six or more egg whites to a skim milkshake each day. If this is continued over a period of months, biotin deficiency is a real possibility. Biotin deficiency does not occur in those who consume an occasional raw egg.

Deficiencies of biotin have also occurred in the past in people who have gastrointestinal surgery and were fed a total diet in a solution via feeding tube. These people need a biotin supplement.

Cases have also been reported of people lacking an enzyme, biotinidase. This enzyme is normally present in pancreatic secretions and is important in releasing biotin from the proteins to which it is attached.

In a classic study some years ago, biotin deficiency was induced (using dried egg white) in four volunteers. After ten weeks, they felt constantly tired, became depressed, developed nausea, loss of appetite, dry scaly skin, muscle aches and pains. Their blood cholesterol levels also rose. All were cured with daily injections of 150 to 300 micrograms of biotin.

Other researchers report symptoms of biotin deficiency to include dermatitis on the face, conjunctivitis, loss of hair and developmental retardation. For those who lack the enzyme biotinidase, deficiency symptoms are different and include seizures, irreversible neurosensory hearing loss and problems with the optic nerve in the eye.

Some people extrapolate from signs of any vitamin deficiency to assume that if they have one or more of the symptoms, it must be due to a deficiency of that vitamin. Baldness is one example. Having read that one symptom of biotin deficiency is loss of hair, some sellers of supplements sell biotin supplements to men who are going bald. It is extremely unlikely that all (or any) of the many men who go bald do so because of biotin deficiency, and there is no evidence that taking biotin can cure baldness.

Similarly, some types of dermatitis are due to biotin deficiency, but most skin rashes and other skin problems have nothing to do with a lack of biotin. Some researchers have given biotin for skin rashes in infants and reported that the rash cleared up. However, rashes come and go, and the only double-blind study to examine the problem found that biotin had no effect.

A biotin deficiency can be diagnosed from an avidin assay. This measures how much avidin added to a sample of blood plasma can be bound, and relates this to the level of biotin present in the plasma. Other methods of measuring biotin are also being developed. Researchers have noted higher levels than normal of odd-chained fatty acids in the plasma of people being fed a total diet via a tube (parenteral nutrition) when the mixture lacked biotin.

Drugs

Long-term use of anti-convulsants (phenobarbital, phenytoin, carbemazepine and primidone) can lead to biotin deficiency. There have been reports of this being severe enough to interfere with the metabolism of amino acids. The drugs appear to interfere with the way cells in the wall of the intestine absorb biotin. Whether a larger intake of biotin in the form of a supplement can overcome this problem is not yet known, but should almost certainly be tried in those taking drugs for many years, such as those with epilepsy.

Excess

There is no data about the effects of excess biotin. Doses of 200 milligrams taken orally, or 20 milligrams by intravenous injection have shown no ill-effects.

Biotin supplements

There is no evidence that a biotin supplement will do any harm, but there are few reports of benefits, with a couple of exceptions.

Anyone who insists on eating large numbers of raw eggs will need a biotin supplement, or preferably be convinced of the foolishness of eating raw eggs. If they continue to eat raw eggs, they will need supplementary biotin given by injection, as the avidin in the raw eggs will bind to any biotin in the intestine, including that from supplements or made by intestinal bacteria.

One study found that women with brittle fingernails who took 2.5 milligrams of biotin a day had a 25 per cent increase in their nail thickness. This study examined the women's nails using electron microscopy. Unfortunately, it did not report on the biotin status of the women before or after the supplement.

Current research findings

Research is still concentrating on the mechanisms by which biotin works, establishing the best method of determining body levels of biotin and also how much is synthesised by bacteria in the intestine.

3

Vitamin C

What it is

What do humans and other primates, guinea pigs, the Indian fruit bat, the red-vented bulbul and a few other birds have in common? The answer is that, unlike other animals and birds, none of them can make their own vitamin C. The problem is almost certainly a genetic defect, but that is of little practical importance since the vitamin can easily be obtained from foods.

Also known as ascorbic acid or ascorbate (and occasionally as ascorbate monoanion), vitamin C is the best known of all the vitamins, probably because of its long—and unproven—association with the common cold.

Vitamin C has an interesting history dating back at least to Vasco da Gama and other sea-going adventurers who first charted world waters from 1497 onwards. Sailors on these trips died from the dreaded disease known as scurvy, a result of vitamin C deficiency.

Captain James Cook's long voyage from 1772 to 1775 was the first to show that sailors could avoid scurvy. Cook gave his crew fresh fruits and vegetables, especially oranges and lemons, whenever they were available. According to some sources, Cook also sprouted wheat grains when other fresh produce was not available.

However, the real credit for rescuing sailors from scurvy should go to James Lind, a Scottish naval surgeon who trialled a variety of foods in his efforts to treat the dreaded scurvy. In 1747, Lind gave some sailors suffering from scurvy, cider or vinegar or sea-water or oranges and lemons. Others were given nutmeg three times a day, a mixture of garlic, mustard seed, balsam and gum myrrh as well as barley water with added tamarind. The citrus fruits worked wonders, the sailors recovered quickly and Lind published his results in 1753. His treatise on the subject was comprehensive, even recognising that scurvy was more likely to affect sailors whose bodies were stressed from excessive alcohol, being wet and cold, and living in crowded dirty conditions. It took some 40 years before the government could be convinced of the need to provide sailors with limes, and from that time on, British sailors were known as 'limeys'.

Even before the discovery of citrus for scurvy, people in Sweden and Russia who could not get fresh fruits and vegetables at certain times of the year knew that pine needles were protective against scurvy. In 1535, Jacques Cartier, a French explorer, helped by native North Americans, revived his ailing crew with the juice of the ameda tree which he found in Newfoundland. Other explorers later died because they failed to identify this tree that would save them as the spruce, a variety of pine.

After its long and eventful history, vitamin C was finally described as a vitamin in 1932, although it had been first isolated from cabbages and oranges in 1928, by a scientist who later received the Nobel Prize for his efforts. A few years later, researchers found that although very small amounts of the vitamin (10 milligrams a day) could cure scurvy, larger quantities were required if the body was under physical stress, including the stress of infection. By 1942, the idea that vitamin C might cure the common cold was tested. The results were negative, but hope persists and many studies have continued. The results have been conflicting, but most have been negative.

Ascorbic acid, as its name suggests, is an acid. If 2000 milligrams is dissolved in 100 millilitres of water, it has a pH of 2.6. When crystallised, the white powder is technically classified as a sugar and is easily oxidised to form a free radical called ascorbate, which is further oxidised to form dehydroascorbic acid. These reactions are reversible, although once dehydroascorbic acid begins its metabolism to other compounds, the steps are no longer reversible. Ascorbic acid is often sold as sodium or calcium ascorbate. These have the same biological activity as ascorbic acid and dissolve easily in water.

What it does

Chemically, ascorbic acid acts as a reducing agent within the body, donating electrons to enzymes or any chemical compounds that are oxidants. It is therefore referred to as an antioxidant.

Once consumed, ascorbic acid is rapidly absorbed from the small intestine. Some goes into the blood plasma and also into white blood cells. Measuring the level in the blood gives an indication of vitamin C status, with the levels in white blood cells being the more accurate.

Ascorbate is a cofactor for eight different enzymes within the body. Three of these need ascorbate for steps in making collagen, the protein that forms the basis of connective tissue and forms a cement-like substance in bones, teeth, gums, blood capillaries, cartilage and connective tissues throughout the body. Another two enzymes need ascorbate to make a substance called carnitine, which is used in the production of energy in muscle cells. Another enzyme uses ascorbate in making norepinephrine (once called noradrenaline), a chemical that carries nerve impulses from one neuron to another and from nerve endings to muscle fibres. And one enzyme needs ascorbate to make a substance called serotonin from the amino acid tryptophan. Serotonin is a neurotransmitter that is present in many body tissues including blood platelets where it acts to constrict the blood vessels and stop bleeding. It is also involved in sleep and may play a role in normal levels of activity, as opposed to hyperactivity.

Part of ascorbate's role as an antioxidant involves protecting DNA from damage. Ascorbate may also prevent oxidation of low density lipoprotein (often referred to as LDL cholesterol or 'bad' cholesterol). Another of its roles is to convert iron to a reduced form (Fe^{2+}) so that it can be absorbed from the intestine. As most of the iron in foods is in the ferric (Fe^{3+}) state, and can only be absorbed in the reduced ferrous (Fe^{2+}) state, vitamin C is vitally important for the absorption of iron from foods. This is a good reason to include a source of vitamin C in each meal, especially for vegetarians whose sources of iron are often poorly absorbed. However, it is potentially a problem for those who have the genetic disorder, haemochromatosis, where too much iron is easily absorbed. Haemochromatosis affects one in 300 people and is especially prevalent in those of Irish descent. Many people with haemochromatosis do not know they have the inherited condition and are therefore unaware that, for them, large doses of vitamin C from supplements are potentially hazardous. One in every eight to ten people carries the gene for haemochromatosis.

Ascorbate has many other functions. It accumulates in certain tissues (for example, the ovaries, testis, pancreas and adrenal cortex of the kidney), although the reasons for the accumulation in these areas are not yet fully understood. The concentration in the adrenal cortex was once thought to be necessary for the role this part of the kidney plays in producing hormones required during stress, including the stress caused by extreme fatigue and infection. However, in cases of scurvy, the adrenal glands continue to produce normal levels of the adrenocortical hormones, so this theory doesn't explain the higher levels of ascorbate found in the adrenal cortex. There is also a high level of ascorbate in the lens and the aqueous humour of the eye (which supplies the lens with its vitamin C).

Vitamin C may also reduce the incidence of cataracts. However, whether this is vitamin C itself, or one of the many carotenoids that occur in foods that are also good sources of vitamin C, is not totally clear. At this stage, the best option seems to be to consume plenty of fruits and vegetables as they contain vitamin C and other substances known to be protective for eyes.

There is certainly some evidence that foods rich in vitamin C may give protection against some cancers. For cancer of the stomach, the vitamin itself may be important in countries where the intake of nitrites is high. These come from preserved, smoked and salted meats and fish and also from the water supply in some areas. Vitamin C acts as a scavenger of nitrite and stops it being converted to nitrosamines, substances known to be involved in causing cancer of the stomach. Even within countries such as Australia, it is probably good practice to have a food rich in vitamin C, such as tomatoes, with preserved meats such as ham, bacon or sausages. Some studies indicate, however, that the intake of vitamin C needs to reach about 1000 milligrams before it begins to function in this way. This point is still unclear.

When some functions of a nutrient are not fully understood, the lack of knowledge is used by some to sell the nutrient as a magic cure for a range of conditions. This has certainly been the case for vitamin C, as it has for several other vitamins.

Large doses of vitamin C were popularised in the 1970s by Linus Pauling, a man who had won two Nobel Prizes—one for Chemistry (in 1954) and the other for Peace (in 1962). Pauling developed an interest in vitamin C after a novelist advised him to try taking large daily doses. Pauling did, felt well and developed fewer colds. He then did some strange calculations and concluded that if early man's diet had consisted solely of plant foods rich in vitamin C, the usual intake would have ranged from 2300 to 12 000 milligrams a day—an amount far greater than the quantities usually recommended. Other researchers who have looked carefully at the total Palaeolithic diet have concluded that the daily vitamin C intake was more like 350 to 400 milligrams. Linus Pauling wrote several popular books about the vitamin, one (which was also revised) devoted to vitamin C and the common cold, another concentrated on using large doses of vitamin C to prevent and cure cancers, and a third recommended megadoses of several vitamins.

The renewed interest in vitamin C that resulted brought millions of dollars to makers of supplements and contributed to this being the most popular vitamin consumed. Unfortunately, many trials of vitamin C have failed to support Pauling's theories.

The common cold

The common cold is not a serious illness but it is responsible for many days of work and quality time lost throughout the world. There have been more than 60 trials of vitamin C and the common cold. The results are diverse and confusing, and at times, experts reviewing the same trials come to different conclusions about the results. However, most trials fail to show that vitamin C has any benefit in reducing the incidence of the common cold. Some say this is because the doses used were not always large enough. But since 1971, there have been at least 21 trials using more than 1000 milligrams of vitamin C—an amount that completely saturates body tissues with the vitamin. Even among these trials, most have shown no reduction in the incidence of colds, but they do show a reduction in the duration and some report less severe symptoms, although this is obviously in the nose of the sufferer.

Linus Pauling appears to have based his conclusions for the efficacy of vitamin C on four trials, some of which reported fewer and shorter colds in children attending skiing camps in the Swiss Alps who took 1000 milligrams of vitamin C a day. As has been noted by other reviewers since, you can't extrapolate from such a group to the general population. However, there are studies showing that vitamin C supplementation reduced the incidence of colds in military troops training hard in Northern Canada and also in long-distance runners, and it is possible that the vitamin has some effect against the common cold virus when the body is under physical stress.

An Australian study (1981) of 95 pairs of identical twins given either vitamin C or a placebo followed the general trend in showing no decrease in incidence of colds with vitamin C, but a reduction in the duration by 19 per cent. This is about as much as any good study has ever shown.

Other variables may also be relevant. For example, a recent study found that there are other aspects relevant to susceptibility to colds. People with a wide social network with good ties to friends and family were much less susceptible to colds than those who were introverted, had increased levels of catecholamines (which indicate that they are stressed in some way), or were poor sleepers. Smoking, abstention from alcohol and having a diet low in fruits and vegetables were also positively related to getting a cold.

Cancer

In the 1970s, Pauling and a Scottish physician, Dr Ewan Cameron, claimed that cancer patients labelled as 'untreatable' survived longer when given vitamin C than a control group. As others have since pointed out, Dr Cameron's patients were labelled as 'untreatable' much earlier in the course of their cancer than the controls, so the results could not be claimed to be due to the vitamin C. To test Pauling's theories, three major controlled trials were conducted by the Mayo Clinic, giving cancer patients 10 000 milligrams of vitamin C. Those getting the vitamin did no better than those on placebo in any of these trials. Several more recent long-term, well-controlled trials of vitamin C supplements for lung cancer, colorectal cancer (the most common internal cancer among men and women in countries such as Australia) and stomach cancer (now rare in most developed countries, but still the most common cancer throughout Asia and some other parts of the world) have all failed to show any effect of the vitamin C.

However, there are now several hundred studies showing that eating more fruits and vegetables is protective against almost all commonly occurring cancers. It is apparently not the vitamin C in these products that is conferring protection, nor the beta carotene or fibre. These vitamins in fruits and vegetables, however, may be important in interacting with the several thousand other components of fruits and vegetables, known collectively as phytochemicals (plant chemicals).

Antioxidant

Great publicity is now being given to compounds that function as antioxidants, and this aspect of vitamin C has become a major reason for its promotion by those marketing supplementary vitamins.

Although vitamin C has antioxidant activity, it is not effective in this respect under all circumstances. For example, although one of its theoretical roles is to prevent the oxidation of low density lipoproteins (LDL, or 'bad' cholesterol), taking vitamin C supplements has not been found to have any effect in reducing LDL levels. It may function as an antioxidant only in conjunction with other antioxidants. For example, vitamin C may be important when the body is using vitamin E as an antioxidant.

Some experts sound a note of warning by reminding us that any compound that acts as an antioxidant can have the opposite effect at high doses when it may function as a pro-oxidant. This point was emphasised recently when a study of healthy volunteers conducted at the University of Leicester in the United Kingdom found that those taking more than 500 milligrams of vitamin C showed adverse DNA changes, compared to those taking a placebo. The authors of this study warn of the fine balance between the body's antioxidant defence system and the undesirable oxidative damage that can give rise to biomolecular damage within the body. It is possible that such damage could predispose towards cancers, rheumatoid arthritis or coronary heart disease. While such effects need to be confirmed before those taking vitamin C supplements become too concerned, other well-known researchers also warn of the danger of large doses of vitamin C from supplements. As large doses (above 500 milligrams a day) have no proven benefits (at least, not when you look only at properly controlled trials), there seems little reason, and some potential pitfalls, in thinking that 'if a little is good, more must be better'—at least for vitamin C from supplements.

How much you need

The recommended dietary intake of vitamin C differs between countries but is generally in the range of 30 to 60 milligrams a day. The RDI in Australia is as follows:

Age	RDI (milligrams)
Breast-fed or bottle-fed	25
7–12 months	30
Boys, 1–15 years	30
Boys, 16–18 years	40
Girls, 1–18 years	30
Men, all ages	40
Women, all ages	30
Pregnancy	60
Lactation	75

These quantities were based on the amount of the vitamin required to prevent scurvy (10 milligrams a day), plus a margin of safety to allow for individual differences in the rate at which the vitamin is used and provide some reserves (although vitamin C is not stored to any extent). This safety margin also takes into account the increased requirements of smokers. The higher quantity recommended for men is to allow for their generally larger body size and the fact that men show lower tissue levels of vitamin C than women. The recommendations for breast-fed infants are based on what they would normally receive from breast milk. Extra vitamin C is not required for these babies, but their mothers need higher levels to cover the losses going into their breast milk. In pregnancy, an intake of 80 milligrams a day is required to prevent falls in maternal levels, as some crosses the placenta to the baby.

There is some dispute over whether these quantities

are sufficient. Many believe that we should aim for tissues to be saturated with vitamin C.

When intake exceeds 130 milligrams a day, unmetabolised ascorbic acid appears in the urine. Some consider that this level represents a desirable intake. Such a level is easily obtainable from food and approximates what the average Australian adult currently consumes.

In some countries, such as the United States, the recommended intake is 60 milligrams a day. Even so, some experts are recommending a higher level of 200 milligrams a day, the quantity that is present if recommended quantities of fruits and vegetables are consumed. They note that cells become saturated with vitamin C if consumption is 100 milligrams a day. They have recommended an intake double this to allow for the possibility of poor absorption from some meals. These experts are *not* recommending supplements of vitamin C.

At 1000 milligrams a day, even the plasma is saturated with vitamin C and this is therefore recommended as the upper safe limit. However, other researchers point out possible problems (see *Excess*) if this quantity is consumed.

Foods contain relatively modest quantities of vitamin C; more than enough, but nothing like the huge doses now appearing in supplements. It seems fair to assume that the amount of vitamin C present in human diets throughout the world is more likely to approximate what humans need. High-dose supplements, which may have a drug-like action, need to be properly evaluated for efficacy and safety before being sold as an unproven cure-all.

Where it is found

Apart from breast milk and offal (liver and kidneys), the major sources of vitamin C are fruits and vegetables. Meat, fish, poultry, eggs, nuts and cheese do not contain vitamin C. Milk contains only small amounts. Raw milk would have a little more but the quantity is still small. The best commonly consumed sources are guavas, citrus fruits, berries and capsicums.

Food	Vitamin C (milligrams)
Fruit	
Apple, 1 medium	10
Apricots, 2 average	14
Apricots, dried, 6	2
Avocado, $\frac{1}{2}$ medium	10
Babaco, $\frac{1}{4}$ medium fruit, 90 g	26
Banana, 1 medium	20
Blackberries, $\frac{1}{2}$ punnet, 100 g	18
Blackcurrants, canned, $\frac{1}{2}$ cup	70
Blackcurrants, fresh, 100 g	200
Canned fruit, average serve	2
Carambola (star fruit), 100 g	35
Cherries, 200 g	30
Cumquats, 4	24
Custard apple, 1 average, 200 g	86
Feijoa, 1 average, 50 g	15
Figs, fresh, 1	3
Fruit salad, average serve, 1 cup	35
Gooseberries, 100 g	40
Grapefruit, $\frac{1}{2}$ medium	48
Grapefruit, canned, $\frac{1}{2}$ cup	38
Grapes, 200 g	12
Guava, 1, 80 g	190
Kiwi fruit, 1 average, 100 g	92

Food	Vitamin C (milligrams)
Lemon, 1 average	72
Lime, 1 average	30
Loganberries, canned, $\frac{1}{2}$ cup	30
Loganberries, fresh, $\frac{1}{2}$ punnet, 100 g	35
Longans, canned, $\frac{1}{2}$ cup	75
Lychee, canned, 6	5
Lychees, raw, 6	35
Mandarin oranges, canned, $\frac{1}{2}$ cup	18
Mango, 1 average, 240 g	66
Mango, green, $\frac{1}{2}$ cup shredded	54
Melon, honeydew, 200 g	36
Melon, rockmelon, 200 g	68
Melon, watermelon, 200 g	16
Mulberries, raw, $\frac{1}{2}$ punnet, 100 g	19
Mulberries, stewed, $\frac{1}{2}$ cup	14
Nashi, 1 medium, 130 g	5
Nectarine, 1 large, yellow flesh, 140 g	6
Nectarines, small, white flesh, 2	35
Orange, 1 medium	75
Passionfruit, 1 average	7
Pawpaw, 1 slice, 150 g	90
Pawpaw, green, $\frac{1}{2}$ cup shredded	18
Peach, 1 average, 140 g	14
Peaches, canned, $\frac{1}{2}$ cup	5
Pear, 1 medium	12
Pepino, 1 average, 100 g	30
Persimmon, 1 average, 95 g	13
Pineapple, 1 slice, 150 g	31
Plums, 2 medium	5
Pomegranate, 1 average, 180 g	25
Prickly pear, 1 average, 90 g	16
Prunes, 6	0
Quince, 1 average, cooked, 200 g	30
Raisins, 50 g	0
Rambutan, 3 medium	47

Food	Vitamin C (milligrams)
Rhubarb, stewed, $\frac{1}{2}$ cup	10
Sultanas, 50 g	0
Strawberries, $\frac{1}{2}$ punnet, 125 g	56
Tamarillo, 1 average, 90 g	14
Tangelo, 1 average, 120 g	34
Juices and drinks	
Apple juice, no added sugar, 1 cup, 250 mL	98
Apple juice, carbonated, 1 cup, 250 mL	12
Blackcurrant cordial, made up, 1 cup, 250 mL	54
Cordial, average strength, 1 cup, 250 mL	2
Grape juice, dark, 1 cup, 250 mL	62
Grapefruit juice, 1 cup, 250 mL	77
Juice drinks (25–35% juice), 1 cup, 250 mL	65
Lemon juice, 1 tablespoon	8
Lime juice, 1 tablespoon	8
Orange juice, prepared, 1 cup, 250 mL	135
Orange & mango juice, 1 cup, 250 mL	172
Pineapple juice, 1 cup, 250 mL	35
Prune juice, canned, $\frac{1}{2}$ cup	0
Tomato juice, canned, 1 cup, 250 mL	50
Vegetable juice, canned, 1 cup, 250 mL	75
Vegetables	
Artichoke, globe, 1 medium	16
Artichoke, Jerusalem, $\frac{1}{2}$ cup cooked	6
Asparagus, steamed, 6 spears	11
Basil, fresh, 1 cup, 30 g	9
Beans, broad, fresh, cooked, 100 g	29
Beans, dried, cooked, 1 cup	0
Beans, frozen, cooked, 100 g	3
Beans, green, cooked, 100 g	13
Beans, snake, cooked, 100 g	22
Bean sprouts, mung, raw, 1 cup	14
Beetroot, cooked, $\frac{1}{2}$ cup	5
Beetroot, canned, $\frac{1}{2}$ cup	0

Food	Vitamin C (milligrams)
Broccoli, cooked, average serve, 100 g	85
Brussels sprouts, cooked, 6	88
Cabbage, green, cooked, 1 cup	55
Cabbage, green, raw, 1 cup	36
Cabbage, red, cooked, 1 cup	50
Capsicum, green, cooked, 50 g	36
Capsicum, green, raw, 100 g	90
Capsicum, cooked, 50 g	70
Capsicum, red, raw, 100 g	170
Capsicum, yellow, raw, 100 g	130
Carrot, mature, raw, 1 medium, 90 g	3
Carrots, cooked, $\frac{1}{2}$ cup	2
Cassava, cooked, 100 g	30
Cauliflower, cooked, 1 cup	75
Celeriac, cooked, $\frac{1}{2}$ cup	11
Celery, raw, 2 celery sticks, 40 g	3
Chilli, long, thin, 1	40
Chilli, mild, 1 medium, 60 g	90
Chilli, small, red, hot, 1	20
Choko, 1 medium, cooked, 120 g	13
Coleslaw, commercial, 100g tub	20
Coriander, fresh, $\frac{1}{2}$ cup	19
Cucumber, Lebanese, raw, 10 slices, 60 g	9
Cucumber, green or apple, 60 g	6
Eggplant, grilled, 100 g	3
Endive, Belgian, raw, average serve, 50 g	9
Fennel, cooked, $\frac{1}{2}$ cup	8
Fennel, raw, $\frac{1}{2}$ cup	10
Kale, cooked, 1 cup	80
Kohl rabi, cooked, $\frac{1}{2}$ cup	65
Kumara, baked, average piece, 120 g	37
Leek, cooked, 1 average, 120 g	29
Lettuce, 4 leaves, 75 g	9
Lotus tubers, 1 piece, 70 g	25
Marrow, cooked, $\frac{1}{2}$ cup	5

Food	Vitamin C (milligrams)
Melon, bitter, 100 g	50
Mint, fresh, 1 tablespoon chopped	3
Mushrooms, raw, 100 g	1
Mustard and cress, $\frac{1}{2}$ cup, 18 g	6
Okra, fried, 75 g	15
Onion, fried in oil, 1 medium	18
Parsley, $\frac{1}{2}$ cup	64
Parsnip, cooked, 1 medium, 150 g	15
Peas, green, frozen, cooked, $\frac{1}{2}$ cup, 80 g	9
Peas, green, raw, $\frac{1}{2}$ cup, 100 g	32
Peas, sugar snap or snow, 1 cup	35
Potato, mashed, 1 cup, 200 g	16
Potato, roast, 1 piece, 100 g	10
Potato, steamed, average serve, 180 g	18
Potato chips, 20 chips	9
Pumpkin, average serve, 120 g	23
Radish, small, red, 2, 30 g	7
Rocket leaves, raw, 50 g	28
Shallots, long green, each	4
Shallots, small brown, cooked, 50 g	9
Silverbeet, cooked, $\frac{1}{2}$ cup	14
Spinach, English, cooked, 100g	16
Spinach, baby, raw, 50 g	14
Spring onion, raw, 2	10
Squash, button, cooked, 2	20
Swede, cooked, $\frac{1}{2}$ cup, 75 g	15
Sweet corn, baby kernels, 100 g	39
Sweet corn kernels, canned or frozen, $\frac{1}{2}$ cup	6
Sweet corn, steamed, 1 cob, 140 g	6
Sweet potato, baked, 1 piece, 125 g	29
Tomato, canned, $\frac{1}{2}$ can, 200 g	22
Tomato puree, canned, $\frac{1}{2}$ cup	48
Tomato, raw, 1 medium, 150 g	26
Turnip, cooked, 100 g	10
Watercress, raw, 1 cup, 40 g	40

Food	Vitamin C (milligrams)
Yam, baked, 1 piece, 120 g	7
Zucchini, cooked, 1 medium, 80 g	19
Other foods	
Breadnut seeds, 100 g	47
Coconut, fresh, 100 g	3
Coconut cream or milk, 100 mL	3
Kidney, cooked, 100 g	3
Jam, 1 tablespoon	2
Liver, cooked, 100 g	17
Liverwurst, 50 g	14
Milk, cow's, regular or low-fat, 1 cup, 250 mL	3
Milk, human, 100 mL	5
Milk, sheep's, raw, 1 cup, 250 mL	12
Milo, 2 teaspoons	11
Potato crisps, 50 g	22

Effect of cooking

Vitamin C is destroyed by heat, light and oxygen and there is no way to prevent some loss during cooking. The best retention of vitamin C occurs with microwave cooking, where losses are extremely small. Steaming or stir-frying preserve much of the vitamin C in vegetables. Losses are much greater when vegetables are boiled, especially if they are placed in a large volume of cold water and brought to the boil. If boiling is inevitable, bring a small quantity of water to the boil, then add the vegetables, cooking only until just tender.

Losses of vitamin C are greater in alkaline conditions. These occur if using copper cooking utensils or if bicarbonate of soda (or baking soda) is added to vegetables. This practice has, thankfully, disappeared, but was once common because it makes green vegetables turn a particularly bright green colour.

There is also some loss of vitamin C during storage of fruits and vegetables. In general, the condition of the produce is a good guide to the levels of vitamins, especially vitamin C, still present. If vegetables have wilted or are damaged, losses are considerable. If vegetables are still crisp and fruits are firm, losses are minimal. It is not correct to say that fruits and vegetables available from supermarkets have lost their vitamins. Modern refrigerated transport and rapid turnover of produce in fruit and vegetable sections mean that much of today's produce may contain more nutrients than occurred in the days when produce was loaded onto the back of a truck and subjected to the sun on its way to and from markets.

Hot storage conditions increase losses of vitamin C and most vegetables (except for onions and potatoes) should be kept in the crisper section of the refrigerator. It is best to use them soon after purchase, but again, the physical condition of fruits and vegetables is a good guide to their retention of vitamin C.

Potatoes are a good source of vitamin C, but the quantities decline with storage time. This was once a greater problem than it is today when different varieties of potatoes that are grown mature throughout the year. In some parts of northern Europe, potatoes are a major contributor to vitamin C intake, although this too is changing as more fresh produce is imported from southern countries during the winter months.

Freezing and canning result in some losses of vitamin C, but modern factory methods have minimised these losses by processing fruits and vegetables soon after picking.

Deficiency

A deficiency is diagnosed by testing blood plasma, or preferably white blood cell levels, of ascorbate.

As described earlier, a deficiency of vitamin C results in scurvy. This condition is now rare, although it occasionally occurs in older people who are unable to get or eat fresh foods, or who cook all foods excessively. The signs of scurvy include gums so swollen that the teeth may not be visible and which bleed at the slightest touch (gums which bleed slightly when brushing teeth are more commonly due to periodontal disease). Haemorrhages also occur in tissues and joints when blood vessels collapse because the collagen that normally supports them breaks down. A common site is just above the knee on the thigh and spontaneous bruising may also occur. Wounds don't heal and old wounds may open up. Osteoporosis also occurs because of collagen breakdown in bone.

Before reaching frank scurvy, signs of deficiency include hypochondriasis, hysteria and depression. Fatigue and lethargy also occur. Each of these are signs of many other physical and psychological problems, and so are not diagnostic on their own. However, anyone who feels constantly tired, and who does not consume fresh fruits and vegetables, should be tested for a deficiency of vitamin C.

Excess

There is no evidence to suggest that eating lots of fruits and vegetables will provide an excess of vitamin C. In those whose intake may be excessive—for example, consuming 20 to 30 typical servings of fruit or vegetables a day—problems of diarrhoea due to excess fibre and sugars that cannot be absorbed efficiently at these levels, or excessive amounts of beta carotene, outweigh any problems from vitamin C.

Vitamin C is not highly toxic, probably because nature has provided several ways for the body to dispose of excess quantities. The human intestine has a limited ability to absorb the vitamin and large quantities (between 1000 and 10 000 milligrams [1 and 10 grams]) leads to diarrhoea. This is a clear but simple indication that the dose is too high. Even with an intake of more than 200 milligrams of vitamin C, the kidneys normally excrete much of the vitamin. When a large dose is given and plasma levels of ascorbate are already high, most of the given dose is rapidly excreted by the kidneys. When excess quantities of vitamin C are taken, more is catabolised within the body.

The supposed benefits of taking large doses of vitamin C, advocated by some and promoted by some companies and individuals selling supplements, are not backed by good evidence. Scientists with no products to sell are warning of the potential for vitamin C to act as a pro-oxidant, in contrast to its valuable antioxidant effects at levels of less than 500 milligrams a day. In the 1970s, when daily doses of several grams of vitamin C were recommended by some, antioxidant and pro-oxidant properties were given much less attention because their full importance, especially in coronary heart disease, had not been recognised at that time.

Vitamin C is acidic and for many years there has been concern that taking large doses of vitamin C and having the excess excreted through the kidneys may increase the chances of developing kidney stones (either oxalate or urate stones). Oxalate is a metabolic by-product of vitamin C metabolism. Whether these stones occur in practice is hotly disputed and may depend on whether the supplement taken is ascorbic acid (which is acidic) or sodium or calcium ascorbate (which are alkaline). High levels of uric acid in the blood have been reported with vitamin C supplements of 3000 milligrams (3 grams) a day. As gout sufferers experience symptoms when their blood uric acid level rises, it makes sense for those with gout to avoid high-dose vitamin C supplements. The way oxalate levels used to be measured after a high dose of vitamin C have been shown to be inaccurate. However, oxalate stones may still occur easily in some people and may still be a good reason for some people to avoid high dose vitamin C supplements. There is no danger with supplements that supply less than 500 milligrams of vitamin C a day.

As described earlier, large doses of vitamin C are also a potential problem for those with haemochromatosis. Those with a rare condition called thalasaemia major, in which there is a severe haemolytic anaemia (with greatly increased production of red blood cells) should also avoid high doses of vitamin C, as they can worsen the condition.

There is also a potential problem that high-dose vitamin C supplements may increase absorption of toxic metals, such as mercury.

High doses of vitamin C are sometimes given intravenously. There is no justification for this and if a doctor or other therapist suggests using injections of vitamin C—especially if the price is high—you should ask a lot of questions and get a second opinion. In people whose bodies do not produce enough of an enzyme called glucose–6-phosphate dehydrogenase, an intravenous dose of vitamin C can cause destruction of red blood cells. As this is a serious condition and there is no evidence for benefits of intravenous vitamin C, the practice is highly questionable. Vitamin C given orally is easily absorbed from the intestine.

There have also been a small number of cases where babies developed scurvy, in spite of an adequate intake of vitamin C from breast milk. These infants' mothers had taken very large doses of vitamin C during their pregnancy, and, presumably, this had induced an extremely high need for the vitamin in their babies. This is unlikely to occur very often but may serve as a warning of the potential danger of large doses of vitamin C during pregnancy.

Vitamin C supplements

From the discussion earlier, a supplement is a poor substitute for eating plenty of fruits and vegetables. However, there is some evidence that a supplement taken at the first signs of the common cold may reduce the duration or severity of the cold. Large quantities of vitamin C are not needed for this purpose, and no more than 500 milligrams a day should be used.

In athletes

Several studies report a lower incidence or shorter duration of the common cold in people exposed to extreme physical activity who take vitamin C supplements. However, there are many communities living in highly mountainous regions where the physical activity levels are extreme. These people seem very fit and healthy, with only moderately low intake of fresh fruits and vegetables to supply vitamin C.

Many studies have given athletes or untrained people 500 to 2000 milligrams of vitamin C a day and then measured their muscular strength, oxygen uptake, training response, endurance and the physical work they produced. In almost all cases, the results—when a training effect is allowed for—have shown no differences between those given the vitamin or a placebo. The only time a slight benefit was seen occurred in a group of athletes who had previous low levels of vitamin C. Once they reached normal blood levels, no further increase in performance was seen.

Strenuous acute exercise increases the levels of ascorbic acid in the blood, in both plasma and white cells. The increase is accompanied by higher levels of plasma cortisol, a hormone released from the adrenal glands. Its significance is not fully understood.

Drugs

Some drugs, such as warfarin (used to 'thin' the blood), aspirin and some anti-depressants may also act differently in the presence of high doses of ascorbic acid. Anyone taking these drugs regularly should check with their doctor before adding vitamin C.

Current research findings

With so much interest in antioxidants and coronary heart disease and also in vitamin supplements and different types of cancer, researchers are continuing studies to work out how vitamin C plays a role. If reading the results of studies, it is important to look at whether a supplement is being used, or whether the study is based on the intake of fruits and vegetables. Some studies report that vitamin C plays a role in some types of cancer, but when you read the details of the study, it is actually fruits and vegetables that are playing a role and the researchers are *assuming* the active agent is vitamin C. As we now know that fruits and vegetables contain literally thousands of antioxidants, and as trials of vitamin C supplements continue to have negative results in preventing problems such as lung cancer or bowel polyps (the forerunner of bowel cancer), most people are realising the need to distinguish between foods and supplements.

4

Vitamin D

What it is

Vitamin D (or more correctly, calciferol) is a generic term and so far, 37 different forms of it have been found. The two major forms are known as vitamin D_2 and vitamin D_3. The compound once called vitamin D_1 was later found to be an impure mixture of several sterols (a combination of fats and alcohol). The vitamin is actually a steroid hormone and plays a vital role in the body's use of calcium.

Vitamin D_2, or ergocalciferol, as it is more properly called, is formed from a reaction between ultraviolet radiation and ergosterol, a sterol found in yeasts and fungi. This is a synthetic form of vitamin D that is used therapeutically and rarely occurs in most animal and plant tissues. It has only a slight difference in its chemistry from other forms of vitamin D and functions as the vitamin within the body.

Vitamin D_3, or cholecalciferol, is the most important

form of vitamin D. It is produced when ultraviolet radiation reacts with a sterol known as 7-dehydrocholesterol. This compound is found in animal fats, including the natural oils in human skin and the oil that birds produce to preen their feathers. One of the essential functions of cholesterol in the human body is to serve as a substrate for making 7-dehydrocholesterol, and its eventual conversion to vitamin D.

Vitamin D was discovered when doctors were searching for a cure for rickets, a crippling bone disease that was once common and still exists in some parts of the world. Well before vitamin D was discovered, cod liver oil was used in Scotland as an effective way to prevent rickets, although no one knew why the fish oil worked. A French doctor spread the word about cod liver oil when he prescribed it extensively in 1860, and its usefulness against rickets was confirmed in 1920 by Sir Edward Mellanby. It was not until the early 1920s that researchers from Britain and Germany showed that a substance in the skin, when subjected to sunlight or ultraviolet irradiation, also gave protection against rickets. By the early 1930s, German researchers had isolated the structure of vitamin D_2. A few years later, the structure and function of the fat-soluble vitamin D_3 became clear and proved to be the previously elusive 'magic' factor in cod liver oil that could prevent rickets.

Vitamin D is different from other vitamins in that as long as we have access to sunlight, there is no dietary requirement for it. However, although we can make this steroid hormone for ourselves, many people do not, usually because of some cultural reason for keeping their skin covered. Many elderly people also do not venture outside into the sunshine, and the fear of skin cancer and use of sunscreens can also mean that some people fail to expose their skin to sunlight.

What it does

Vitamin D is essential for the body to use calcium. It starts by promoting the absorption of calcium from the intestine, then helps control the amount of calcium that goes from the blood to the bones and vice versa.

The first stage in the production of vitamin D is that sunlight acts on 7-dehydrocholesterol, converting it to vitamin D_3. (Alternatively, vitamin D_3 can be obtained from foods in which it occurs naturally or to which it has been added.) Vitamin D_3 is called a pro-hormone and is metabolised in the liver to 25-hydroxy-cholecalciferol, which then circulates in the blood. The kidneys then enter the picture and convert 25-hydroxycholecalciferol to two other forms of vitamin D_3, the major one being 1-alpha, 25-dihydroxy-cholecalciferol. This active form of vitamin D_3, made in the kidneys, functions as a hormone and has ten times the activity level of vitamin D_3 itself. It also acts more quickly and works with two other hormones—parathyroid hormone and calcitonin—to regulate the metabolism of calcium and phosphorus within the body.

In the 1960s, researchers also found that once vitamin D had been converted to its active form, vitamin D_3, specific proteins were synthesised to transport vitamin D_3 and all its metabolites to the various target organs.

The kidney exerts great control over the different forms of vitamin D. When blood levels of the active form of D_3 are low, the kidney produces more and when the levels in the blood are high, it produces less.

Vitamin D_3 in its active form helps calcium absorption from the intestine by causing a specific calcium-binding protein to be made in the cells lining the small intestine. Working with parathyroid hormone, the active form of D_3 also acts on bone to release some calcium to the blood. As a follow-up, it then helps the absorption of phosphate by a separate mechanism. As well, there are nuclear receptors for the active form of vitamin D_3 in most tissues throughout the body. These regulate the metabolism of many specific genes and proteins within the body.

The most studied function of vitamin D is with calcium metabolism. The level of calcium in the blood is vitally important for nerves and muscles to function properly. If the level falls, the parathyroid glands produce more parathyroid hormone which stimulates enzymes in the kidneys to increase production of the active form of vitamin D_3. This then mobilises calcium from bone to bring the level of calcium in the blood back to normal. When there is enough calcium in the blood, the kidneys stop producing the active form of D_3.

Vitamin D also plays a role in the metabolism of phosphorus and is involved in preventing excessive cell division in the body. Apart from bone, tissues that rely on vitamin D include the kidneys, intestine, breast tissue, the pancreas, the pituitary gland, placenta, skin and blood-forming cells.

How much you need

The exact amount of vitamin D required has never been precisely defined, mainly because the amount that comes when sunlight acts on the skin is difficult to measure and also because a dietary source is not usually necessary. However, in areas of the world where the winters are so cold that the whole body is covered by clothing, and in parts where women are veiled and do not expose their skin to the sun, vitamin D must be obtained from the diet. The very real dangers of skin cancer have also meant that some people protect their skin from sunlight with hats and clothing, or use sunscreen lotions that screen out ultraviolet light. There is also some evidence that extreme pollution in some cities stops the ultraviolet radiation reaching the skin. If these conditions apply all the time, and the body can't make its own vitamin D, the vitamin must then be supplied from the diet, like other vitamins.

Vitamin D can be stored in the body for long periods. The body's very limited ability to cope with excess amounts of vitamin D taken orally has led to upper safe limits for oral intake being set in some countries.

The activity of vitamin D is defined as 1 microgram of cholecalciferol = 40 International Units (IU) of vitamin D. Most countries that have set an allowance for a reasonable intake, have taken 5 or 10 micrograms (or 20–40 IU) a day as their recommendation. In Australia, no recommended dietary intake has been set, as the vitamin is not required from the diet. In the United States and many other countries where exposing skin to sunlight is not practical or possible, the intake is set at 7.5 micrograms for the first six months of life, 10 micrograms a day until adult life and 5 micrograms a day after that. During pregnancy, the recommended daily level is 10 micrograms (or 40 IU).

Studies have recently shown that the level of vitamin D_3 increases during pregnancy. This is almost certainly to prevent excessive loss of calcium from the mother.

The amount of sunlight on skin for adequate production of vitamin D is usually about one to two hours a week. This quantity will vary to some extent, depending on the quality of the sunlight. If this is not possible, dietary sources of vitamin D may need consideration.

Where it is found

Vitamin D is found naturally in oily fish and the oils from their livers. The fish get their vitamin D by eating plankton which are near enough to the surface of the sea to be exposed to sunlight. There are small quantities in eggs, cream and butter. In some countries, low-fat milks and some margarines have vitamin D added. A few cereals, fortified yoghurt drinks and soy beverages also have added vitamin D. These values change from time to time as products are reformulated, so it is necessary to check the labels of foods before relying on foods fortified with vitamin D.

Vitamin D does not occur in nuts, avocado, vegetable oils or other plant-based foods. Cakes made with butter and eggs may contain some vitamin D. Cheese sauces, egg mayonnaise and dishes made with cheese sauce, such as lasagne will contain some vitamin D.

Food	Vitamin D (micrograms)
Dairy products and eggs	
Butter, 1 tablespoon, 20 g	0.15
Cheese, average, 50 g	0.13
Cottage cheese, 50 g	0.01
Cream, 50 mL	0.14
Goat's milk, 1 cup, 250 mL	0.28

Food	Vitamin D (micrograms)
Milk, fat-reduced, 1 cup, 250 mL	0.03
Milk, fat-reduced, with added vitamin D, 1 cup, 250 mL	3.75
Milk, full-cream, 1 cup, 250 mL	0.08
Milk, human, 100 mL	0.04
Milk, skim, 1 cup, 250 mL	0
Milk, sheep's, 1 cup, 250 mL	0.45
Yoghurt, regular, plain or fruit, 200 g	0.08
Egg, hen, 1	0.88
Egg white	0
Offal	
Liver, lamb's fry, cooked, 100 g	0.50
Liver, chicken, cooked, 100 g	0.20
Liver, calf, cooked, 100 g	0.30
Liver, pig, cooked, 100 g	1.10
Liver, ox, cooked, 100 g	1.10
Fish	
Cod liver oil, 1 tablespoon	42.00
Herring, grilled, 100 g	25.00
Herring, raw, 100 g	22.50
Kippers, cooked, weighed with bones, 100 g	13.50
Mackerel, cooked, weighed with bones, 100 g	15.40
Mackerel, smoked, 100 g	8.00
Pilchards, canned, 100 g	8.00
Salmon, canned, 100 g	12.50
Sardines, canned, 100 g	7.50
Tuna, canned in brine, drained, 100 g	4.00
Tuna, canned in oil, drained, 100 g	5.80
Miscellaneous	
Horlicks powder, 2 teaspoons	0.20
Margarine, fortified with vitamin D, 20 g, 1 tablespoon	1.10
Ovaltine powder, 2 teaspoons	0.21

Effect of cooking

There is some loss of vitamin D in cooking (up to 40 per cent from some foods), but generally the vitamin is stable to heat and does not diminish greatly with storage.

Deficiency

As discussed briefly, a lack of vitamin D causes rickets, a disease where growing bones do not absorb calcium properly and become soft and misshapen as a result. When the disease occurs in adults, it is known as osteomalacia. It is common in women in Middle Eastern countries where their clothing covers the whole body, including a veil over the face, so that sunlight cannot produce the precursor of vitamin D.

Normally, bone growth occurs in the band of cartilage lying between the shaft of a bone and the knobbly part on its end. New cartilage forms continuously and the old cartilage degenerates, with capillaries and new bone cells (called osteoblasts) forming bony tissue within it, taking up more calcium in the process. Growth ceases when no more new cartilage forms and the shaft bone meets and fuses with the end part of the bone.

Vitamin D is essential for the degeneration of the old cartilage. With insufficient quantities of the vitamin, the gap between the shaft and the knobbly end of the bone widens and bony tissue in the space becomes irregular. Little calcification takes place, causing growing bones to become distorted and soft. The layer covering the outer surface of bones also fails to accumulate a normal amount of calcium. These changes produce rickets (from the Anglo-Saxon word *wrikken*, meaning 'twisted'). In adults, the bones have stopped growing and a lack of vitamin D results in bones becoming soft from demineralisation. Hard bone is replaced with soft bony tissue. The spine, pelvis and legs are especially affected.

Both rickets and osteomalacia are known as diseases of poverty and darkness. Rickets can also occur in infants of low birth weight born to mothers who themselves are deficient in vitamin D and therefore have only low levels in their milk. Neither disease should occur anywhere in the world, because the knowledge to prevent them is available and means to fix them is cheap.

A lack of vitamin D is one factor involved in osteoporosis—a condition that is common and increasing rapidly in Western countries as people live longer. Studies of elderly people show lower than normal levels of vitamin D_3 than in younger adults. This is especially likely to be the case in elderly people who are not able to go outside, but it is also possible that elderly people may have a reduced ability to convert 7-dehydrocholesterol in the skin to vitamin D_3. Several trials in which elderly people were given vitamin D supplements found a reduced incidence of bone fractures compared with others given a placebo. However, these studies were done in Finland or in nursing home residents. Whether similar results would occur with older people who are still active and have access to sunlight is not yet known.

Drugs

Some anti-epileptic drugs and sedatives, such as phenobarbitone, accelerate the metabolism of vitamin D and, if used long term, can increase the chances of developing rickets and osteomalacia.

Excess

Vitamin D is the most toxic of all vitamins in that a long-term daily dose five times the usually recommended intake, can be toxic. Excess vitamin D does not occur from sunlight acting on skin, for several reasons. Too much sunlight on skin induces more pigmentation and this prevents conversion of the pro-vitamin 7-dehydrocholesterol to vitamin D_3. As a further feedback precaution, as mentioned earlier, when levels of vitamin D_3 are high, the kidneys convert less of it to the active form.

An excess of vitamin D can arise from taking supplements or excessive quantities of foods fortified with vitamin D or from cod liver oil. People in countries of northern Europe are justified in taking cod liver oil, although more is not better. But in countries such as Australia, where there is ample sunshine, cod liver oil is not recommended.

The usual reason for taking cod liver oil is not for its vitamin D content, but because it is also an excellent source of omega 3 fatty acids. These are available from commercial fish oil preparations, from which the vitamin has been removed. Some people also take cod liver oil for its vitamin A, but again, the levels are much too high for anyone whose diet also contains enough of this vitamin. Since vitamin A taken during pregnancy, even in relatively low doses, can cause birth deformities, cod liver oil should not be taken by pregnant women. In fact, there is no justification, and many reasons against anyone in countries such as Australia taking this fish oil.

There have been reports of vitamin D poisoning from high consumption of milk products fortified with extra vitamin D. Symptoms include loss of appetite, nausea, vomiting, muscular weakness, joint pains, intense thirst and frequent urination. The bones become demineralised and the person is generally disoriented. If the excess intake continues, calcium is deposited in soft tissues such as the lungs and kidneys, and death results.

The effects of an excess intake of vitamin D are much higher if the supplement used contains 1-alpha, 25-dihydroxycholecalciferol, the active form of vitamin D_3. The normal feedback mechanisms by the kidneys to control the levels of this form of the vitamin are bypassed if supplements containing this substance are used.

Vitamin D supplements

A vitamin D supplement should only ever be taken in cases where levels are shown to be low, using appropriate medical analysis of blood levels.

Many brands of vitamin D supplements contain the active form of vitamin D_3. Those containing high quantities (50 to 1000 micrograms a day) should only be used under medical supervision for treatment of established vitamin D deficiency. This may occur in hypothyroidism or in various kidney diseases.

When active forms of vitamin D are used for treating osteoporosis, the quantity used is usually of the order of 0.25 to 1 microgram a day. This level is unlikely to have any toxicity.

Supplements of vitamin D are not recommended for general use. It is better to expose the skin to sunlight for short periods.

In athletes

There is no evidence that athletes need extra vitamin D. One study reported that athletes involved in weight training had higher levels of vitamin D in the blood. This was almost certainly because their exercise was increasing calcium deposition in bone and the body was simply responding normally and converting more vitamin D to the active form. There is no indication that these or other athletes benefit from vitamin D supplements and no rationale to recommend that athletes should use them.

Current research findings

Much of the current research into vitamin D concerns its role in osteoporosis. Initial results show that vitamin D helps reduce bone fractures in elderly people, but there have not yet been trials to see if extra time spent in sunlight may be as valuable as a supplement.

Researchers are also looking at a possible role for vitamin D in treating leukaemia and cancers of the breast, colon and prostate gland. It may also play a part in preventing rejection of transplanted organs.

Some studies from the Netherlands have shown that elderly men who lacked vitamin D had impaired glucose tolerance. As this is associated with diabetes, the relationship is being studied further.

In Finland, where vitamin D intake is low and colorectal cancer incidence is high, researchers have found that male smokers who get cancer of the rectum have low levels of 25-hydroxycholecalciferol. The significance of this is not currently known but may deserve further study.

5

Vitamin E

What it is

Vitamin E was first discovered during the major years of vitamin research in the 1920s. Two Californian researchers found that vegetable oils could correct infertility in rats which occurred when their diet consisted of casein, cornflour, lard, butter and yeast. It was not until 1936 that the same researchers finally isolated and identified vitamin E from wheat-germ oil. They called it tocopherol, from two Greek words, *tokos* meaning 'child', and *pherein* meaning 'carry'. The vitamin was synthesised in Switzerland and in the United States in 1938.

Vitamin E is a group of eight related compounds called tocopherols and tocotrienols. In appearance, tocopherols are yellow and oily. They have been designated as alpha (α), beta (β), gamma (γ) and delta (δ), depending on slight differences in their chemical structure. For each of the tocopherols, there are eight possible compounds containing the same number of atoms, arranged slightly differently (called isomers). The most abundant of these in natural foods is called *d*-alpha-tocopherol or *d*-α-tocopherol. This is sometimes called natural vitamin E and is the most biologically active form. Vitamin E activity is expressed in terms of this isomer.

When vitamin E is made in the laboratory, an equal number of each of the tocopherol isomers forms. Synthetic vitamin E was once called *dl*-α-tocopherol (and this term is still found on most supplements), but is now more correctly known as all-racemic α-tocopherol. This newer term reflects the fact that the synthetic tocopherol consists of substances that are dextro-rotatory (*d*) and laevo-rotatory (*l*) in the way they polarise light.

The tocotrienols (α, β, γ and δ), have a slightly different structure and until recently were considered to be of less significance than the tocopherols. However, the biological activity of some compares favourably with some of the tocopherols and they are now a subject of major research.

All forms of vitamin E are fat-soluble and are found in conjunction with fats in foods, although the actual quantity of fat present need not necessarily be large, as is the case with vitamin E found in vegetables. Some fat is required for absorption of vitamin E from the intestine, however, and there is a danger that an obsession with minimal fat intake could lead to lower levels of vitamin E being absorbed. Vitamin E also usually occurs in foods containing fats.

Vegetables have a little vitamin E, although less than fatty foods such as seeds, nuts and oils. Eating some type of oil or other fat with vegetables will increase absorption of their vitamin E.

Vitamin E is sometimes described as milligrams of alpha tocopherol equivalents and sometimes as International Units (IU) of vitamin E. To make comparisons between these, the usual equivalence is taken as 1 IU = 0.67 milligrams of alpha tocopherol equivalents. To convert IU to milligrams, you therefore multiply the number by 0.67. Thus 100 IU = 67 milligrams of alpha tocopherol equivalents. Occasionally, you see advice to multiply by 0.74, but most authorities use 0.67.

What it does

Vitamin E functions in the body as an antioxidant. It is present in the membranes around every body cell where it helps prevent oxidation of polyunsaturated fats in the membrane. Vitamin E carries out this function by acting as a scavenger of free radicals. These are produced continuously as we use oxygen and they have the potential to damage the polyunsaturated fats present in the membranes around every cell. This is one of the reasons why the body needs vitamin E and other antioxidants.

Oxidative damage also occurs to some of the protein constituents of membranes and vitamin E may help prevent this too. There is also some evidence that vitamin E may prevent damage to DNA and RNA (ribonucleic acid). In this role, there has been some hope that the vitamin may have anti-cancer activity, since damage to DNA contributes to the initiation stage of many cancers.

When the tocopherol molecule reacts with a free radical, it is converted to a tocopheroxyl radical. This can be converted back to tocopherol by vitamin C or a reducing substance produced by the body called glutathione (a tripeptide of the amino acids glutamic acid, cysteine and glycine), present in the plasma. Glutathione becomes oxidised itself in this process and is an important part of the body's natural defence system. Ubiquinol, another antioxidant produced by the body, may also be able to regenerate tocopherols.

For many years there was widespread acceptance that vitamin E was important, but few specific mechanisms for its suspected actions were known. More recently there has been an explosion of research into vitamin E, some of it generated by those funded by companies hoping to sell vitamin E supplements. However, it is fair to say that some of the research is independently funded.

The evidence for the usefulness of large doses of vitamin E is still controversial and specific proof for many of the suspected roles is hard to come by. That does not seem to hinder sales and among single vitamins, vitamin E continues to rate well, especially with women. The fact that few people know which foods contain this vitamin probably helps sales of vitamin E pills.

Cancer

Some recent functions proposed for vitamin E include its involvement in the body's immune response, through its involvement in preventing damage to DNA and RNA. It is hoped that it may have important effects in preventing various cancers. This can only be proved by long-term clinical trials, and five major trials looking at cancers of the lung and bowel have not shown benefits. Studies currently in progress may yield more information, although with no evidence in favour and five trials showing no results, only an optimist would hold much hope of finding anything dramatic in this aspect of using vitamin E.

Cardiovascular disease

Much of the emphasis on vitamin E has concerned its role in coronary heart disease. This connection strengthened as a large body of evidence showed that low density lipoprotein (LDL or 'bad' cholesterol) only really becomes harmful when it is oxidised. In this oxidised form, LDL damages the cells in the arteries and generates foam cells laden with fat. These represent one of the earliest stages of atherosclerosis in which fatty deposits build up in the arteries, reducing the size of the artery, making the heart pump harder to get blood through the narrowed blood vessel and acting as an ideal site for a clot to form and cause a heart attack. The theory is that vitamin E, having antioxidant properties, will prevent the oxidation of LDL and thus the fat deposits in the arteries.

The evidence for vitamin E being useful to protect against coronary heart disease is more hopeful. Test tube studies show that vitamin E can prevent LDL accumulating in foam cells. There are also studies in cells showing that vitamin E can decrease oxidative changes. And many observational (epidemiological) studies have shown that populations and individuals with a higher intake of vitamin E have a lower incidence of coronary heart attacks.

The largest studies usually used as proof of the usefulness of vitamin E were the Health Professionals Study (39 910 men) and the Nurses Health Study (87 245 women), both of which reported decreased risk of coronary heart disease in those who had the highest blood levels of vitamin E. The risk was 40 per cent lower in the men and 34 per cent lower in the women with the highest blood levels. A closer inspection showed that most of the difference occurred in those who took vitamin E as a supplement. Of these people, 41 per cent of the women and 37 per cent of the men who used at least 100 IU (67 milligrams) for at least two years had a reduced risk. Of course, such studies do not prove that vitamin E was necessarily supplying the protection, because those who take vitamin E supplements for many years may well practise other behaviours that are protective against heart disease. But it seems a hopeful area for study.

In other studies from Finland (12 000 subjects), the Netherlands (10 523 subjects), however, there has been no consistent association between vitamin E concentration in the blood and risk of death from coronary heart disease. The same findings were reported from the large EURAMIC study conducted in nine European centres and in Israel. Low levels of vitamin E in adipose (fat) tissue were not associated with any increased risk of heart attack. Another large study of 34 000 post-menopausal women in Iowa found no evidence of any protection from taking supplements of vitamin E, although they reported a reduced risk of death from coronary heart disease in women who consumed more vitamin E from food sources.

A fifteen-year study of men in the Netherlands found no association between the intake of vitamin C or vitamin E and risk of stroke. The researchers did report that those men who had the highest intake of flavonoids, another type of antioxidant, had the lowest risk of stroke.

The MONICA study of 16 European population groups showed that those who had higher levels of vitamin E in their blood had a lower risk of coronary heart disease. These levels were much lower than those that result from high-dose supplements and may either reflect a value for foods sources of vitamin E or some other virtues of the foods that contain this vitamin.

Other studies have given vitamin E supplements of 60, 200, 400, 800 or 1200 IU a day (40, 134, 268, 536 or 804 milligrams) for eight weeks and measured the susceptibility of LDL to oxidise in blood samples taken from those using supplements. With higher levels of vitamin E, there was less oxidation of LDL, but only if they took at least 400 IU a day (268 milligrams).

In an Australian study, there was no difference in oxidation of LDL when supplements of 500, 1000 or 1500 IU a day (335, 670 or 1005 milligrams) were given for six weeks.

Some studies have used lower doses of vitamin E of 25 IU a day (17 milligrams) or 150 IU a day (100 milligrams) for one week and then 300 IU a day (200 milligrams) for three weeks, and have also reported slower rates of oxidation of LDL. One study in people with diabetes reported lower levels of blood peroxides (substances that increase the risk of coronary heart disease) with a supplement of 100 IU (67 milligrams). The dose required to prevent oxidation eventually occurring is unclear in view of the conflicting results so far.

The usefulness of vitamin E in preventing or curing cardiovascular disease obviously is not completely proven. The only real proof of the usefulness of taking supplementary vitamin E can come from clinical trials where supplements and all dietary sources of this and other vitamins, and other antioxidants, are monitored, along with fatal and non-fatal heart attacks and strokes.

One study in Cambridge (the Cambridge Heart Antioxidant Study or CHAOS), gave 2002 people with proven evidence of atherosclerosis in their coronary arteries a daily supplement of natural vitamin E. Subjects took either 400 IU (268 milligrams a day) for one year or 800 IU (536 milligrams a day) for two years. Non-fatal heart attacks were reduced after 200 days of the study, but total deaths from cardiovascular disease overall was slightly higher in the group taking extra vitamin E. The difference was not significant but was greatest in those taking 800 IU. The reduction in non-fatal heart attacks was greater in those taking the lower dose of vitamin E. This study does not show benefits for vitamin E supplements, and may ring alarm bells about high-dose supplements.

In the ATBC (Alpha-Tocopherol, Beta-Carotene Cancer Prevention Study) in Finland (see *Beta carotene*), those given 50 milligrams of vitamin E for up to eight years had fewer deaths due to ischaemic heart disease and ischaemic stroke, but more deaths due to haemorrhagic stroke. While this could simply mean that if you don't die of one condition, you are more likely to get another, it does suggest caution before we sing the praises of vitamin E supplements.

Some experts believe that the levels of vitamin E used may not always be large enough to see any result. Others maintain that combinations of beta carotene, vitamin C and vitamin E would give more consistent results, but only vitamin E has shown any effect in decreasing LDL oxidation in blood samples.

When vitamin E appears to be effective in doses that

could never be found in natural foods, it is acting as a drug. As such, it needs proper research for efficacy, side effects and safety, as we would expect and demand for any drug. It is also important to consider whether convincing some people that a high-dose vitamin supplement will help prevent coronary heart disease may reduce their compliance with other protective and proven actions such as lowering dietary saturated fat and increasing exercise.

In the Iowa women's study referred to earlier, there appeared to be a 25 per cent increase in risk of death from coronary heart disease in women who took supplements containing 100 to 250 IU (67 to 168 milligrams) of vitamin E and a 9 per cent increase in those taking higher doses. While this is no more proof than the observations of benefits from previous studies, it does flag the fact that more research is needed before advising large doses of vitamin E.

Many more studies are in progress but at this stage the results can only be described as equivocal. Perhaps the most disturbing aspect of vitamin E having a possible antioxidant effect in preventing oxidation of LDL cholesterol, is the dramatic differences in the quantity claimed to be effective in different studies. Some indicate that the dose needs to be above 800 IU (536 milligrams) to show any effect, whereas others report adverse effects from so much and benefits from much lower doses.

Vitamin sellers are hopeful that future research results may support a role for vitamin E in age-related macular degeneration of the eye; decreased cataract risk; preventing diabetes in susceptible people (who are also at high risk of coronary heart disease); protecting sperm in smokers (who have lower levels of vitamin E in their sperm than non-smokers); protecting lung tissue from oxidative damage in those with cystic fibrosis increasing bone minerals (experiment so far in chickens); delaying progress in Alzheimer's disease; increased rate of wound healing (as occurs in animals given vitamin E); improving the immune response in the elderly.

At this stage, there is some support for most of these possible functions. However, studies are also showing no significant correlation between vitamin E and cognitive function in older people. Men with prostate cancer or lung cancer have low blood levels of vitamin E, but whether this is a cause or result of the cancer is not known. In the ATBC trial in Finland, male smokers given 50 milligrams of vitamin E a day had a 23 per cent lower incidence of prostate cancer. As this was not a trial for prostate cancer, the results need to be backed-up from other studies. No association has generally been found between vitamin E supplements and risk of breast cancer, although one Italian study reported a reduced intake of vitamin E in women with breast cancer compared with a control group. This study asked women about their intake of a restricted range of foods, and this limits the usefulness of the information.

Among the confusing studies about diet and cataracts, the best evidence almost certainly shows protection from a high intake of fruits and vegetables. It may not be valid to extrapolate from this to assume that it is the vitamin E (or the vitamin C or beta carotene) in these foods that is responsible, especially since they also contain many thousands of other compounds, at least some of which (carotenoids other than beta carotene) have been found to be highly relevant to cataracts.

Vitamin E used to be described as 'the vitamin in

search of a disease'. Such a tag is no longer appropriate, but it is one of the more perplexing nutrients because so many studies fail to find any significant effect between the amount of vitamin E that can be obtained from a well-chosen diet and disease conditions. Most notable effects have only been seen when very large doses of vitamin E have been used, usually given as alpha tocopherol. In the extremely large doses that are sometimes effective (and sometimes are not), vitamin E is obviously functioning in a way that is different from its normal nutrient role.

Even with extremely large therapeutic doses of vitamin E, the effects are inconsistent. For example, in stimulating immune response in elderly people, a dose of 200 milligrams produced favourable results that were not found with 60 or 800 milligram doses.

One report that a dose of 100 milligrams of vitamin E was needed to normalise tissue vitamin E levels in people with cystic fibrosis was at least understandable in that the vitamin may be poorly absorbed in this condition. A 15 milligram dose had no effect.

A glimmer of hope for sales of vitamins C and E occurred with a recent study showing that large doses— 1000 milligrams of vitamin C and 800 IU (536 milligrams) vitamin E—taken with a fatty meal, prevented the usual changes seen in the diameter of arteries after such a meal. After a low-fat meal, with an equally high number of kilojoules, the vitamins had no effect. While the authors are careful to point out that their findings are preliminary, this is an obvious selling point for vitamin companies. Dietitians might be somewhat anxious, because there is no suggestion that taking these large quantities of vitamins will remove other risk factors associated with meals high in fat, especially saturated fats.

Other forms of vitamin E

Until recently, the significance of carotenoids, other than beta carotene, was ignored. Because other carotenoids had a low rate of conversion to vitamin A, they were usually dubbed 'non nutrients' and assumed to be fairly useless. The latest research, especially into the value of fruits and vegetables in preventing cancer, shows the folly of having ignored components of food, just because their function was not understood and did not fit in with the prevailing interest of the time (which was how well they could be converted to vitamin A). Vitamin C and beta carotene in fruits and vegetables now appear to be much less potent in preventing cancer than other components of these foods.

Some similar situation could possibly exist with other forms of vitamin E. Alpha tocopherol is described as the most bioactive type; β-tocopherol is described as having up to 50 per cent activity, γ-tocopherol as having 10 to 35 per cent activity, δ-tocopherol as having only 3 per cent activity. Among the tocotrienols, α-tocotrienol has 50 per cent activity, β-tocotrienol as having 5 per cent activity, while the potency of the other two tocotrienols is less clear. In general, only α-tocopherol is regarded as important and the other forms are largely ignored, even though they are the predominant forms in natural foods.

It is possible that other forms of vitamin E may be less effective as sources of vitamin E, just as the many other carotenoids are not effective as sources of vitamin A. However, as the other carotenoids have their own role, so too the other forms of vitamin E may yet be found to have value, although this is not often considered at present. At this stage, such statements are pure conjecture, but when nature provides a range of compounds, there is often a reason for their existence.

The β, γ and δ forms of tocopherol are certainly better antioxidants in the test tube, so it seems strange that they are so often ignored. Food composition tables may also give an inaccurate estimate of the total vitamin E level in foods, since the different types are discounted according to their level of activity when compared with α-tocopherol.

The type of vitamin E and the relevant role it plays may be important determinants of the usefulness of vitamin E.

Absorption

Between 20 and 50 per cent of dietary α- and γ-tocopherol is normally absorbed. The process is similar to the way fats are absorbed. Bile acids from the liver are released into the intestine and help carry the vitamin E across into cells lining the intestine. Enzymes released from the pancreas and intestine are involved too. Anything that prevents normal digestion and absorption of dietary fat will also adversely effect absorption of vitamin E. This includes some liver diseases and conditions such as cystic fibrosis.

Vitamin E is initially carried in the blood in chylomicrons (combinations of protein and fat), but is then released to tissues or carried on high-density lipoproteins (HDL, or 'good' cholesterol). This occurs more in females. In males, vitamin E is carried by low-density lipoproteins (LDL, or 'bad' cholesterol). Normal blood plasma levels of α-tocopherol for adults range from 5 to

20 micrograms per millilitre. Children have lower levels and babies born prematurely have the lowest levels.

Vitamin E goes to the liver, but is rapidly turned over and very little is stored in there. Some tocopherol accumulates slowly in fatty tissue but most is stored in the muscles. Turnover rates are rapid in the plasma, liver, lung and kidney. It stays longer in muscle, brain, spinal cord, heart and testes in males.

How much you need

The recommended dietary intake of vitamin E has been difficult to establish because so few cases of deficiency are seen. Because the amount of vitamin E needed depends on the amount of polyunsaturated fat consumed, the recommended intake has been increased since polyunsaturated fat intake has increased.

Age	RDI (milligrams alpha tocopherol equivalents)
Breast-fed, 0–6 months	2.5
Bottle-fed, 0–6 months	4.0
7–12 months	4.0
Children, 1–3 years	5.0
Children, 4–7 years	6.0
Children, 8–11 years	8.0
Boys, 12–15 years	10.5
Boys, 16–18 years	11.0
Girls, 12–15 years	9.0
Girls, 16–18 years	8.0
Men, all ages	10.0
Women, all ages	7.0
Pregnancy	7.0
Lactation	9.5

In the past, the recommended dietary intake for adults was 5 milligrams, but this was when the diet had more saturated and less polyunsaturated fats. The recommended intake for women is lower because they generally eat less, including less polyunsaturated fat. The difference for bottle-fed babies is because many formula milks contain more polyunsaturated fats than breast milk.

Where it is found

The best source of vitamin E is wheat germ, or, if you have a good fresh supply, wheat-germ oil. Other good sources include avocado, vegetable oils, seeds, nuts and wholegrains. Some breads and cereals have added vitamin E, although this may not provide the whole range of types of vitamin E.

Food	Vitamin E (milligrams)
Breads, grains and cereals	
Barley, wholegrain, $\frac{1}{4}$ cup raw, 45 g	0.4
Biscuits, sweet, 2	0.6
Bran, wheat, 1 tablespoon, 8 g	0.2
Bread, rye, 1 slice, 50 g	0.6
Bread, white, 1 slice, 30 g	trace
Bread, wholemeal, 1 slice, 30 g	0.1
Cake, chocolate, average slice, 110 g	3.0
Cake, rich fruit, average slice, 100 g	2.3
Crackers, wholemeal, 4, 40 g	0.6
Flour, white, 1 cup, 125 g	0.4
Flour, wholemeal, 1 cup, 130 g	1.8
Oats, rolled, raw, $\frac{1}{2}$ cup, 50 g	0.9
Oats, porridge, cooked, average bowl	0.8
Pasta, egg noodles, fried, 1 cup, 170 g	4.5
Pasta, wholemeal, cooked, 1 cup, 180 g	trace

Food	Vitamin E (milligrams)
Pastry, average piece in one-crust pie	1.4
Rice, brown, cooked, 1 cup, 180 g	0.5
Scone, plain, 1 average	0.7
Scone, wholemeal, 1 average	1.4
Soy flour, full-fat, 1 cup, 150 g	2.2
Wheat germ, 1 tablespoon, 10 g	2.2
Dairy products	
Cheese, average of main varieties, 50 g	0.3
Cheese, cottage, 50 g	trace
Cheese, ricotta, 50 g	trace
Cream, 50 g	0.4
Cream, clotted, 50 g	0.7
Ice cream, 100 mL	0.1
Milk, cow's, regular, 1 cup	0.2
Milk, cow's, skim, 1 cup	0
Milk, goat's, 1 cup	trace
Milk, human, breast, 100 mL	0.3
Milk, human, colostrum, 100 mL	1.3
Milk, sheep's, 1 cup	0.3
Yoghurt, natural or fruit, low-fat, 200 g	0
Yoghurt, natural or fruit, regular, 200 g	0.1
Yoghurt, soy, 200 g	3.0
Meat, poultry and eggs	
Bacon, grilled, 2 rashers, 60 g	0.1
Beef or veal, cooked, average serve, 150 g	0.4
Chicken, average serve, 150 g	0.1
Chicken curry, Indian, average serve	5.6
Egg, hen, boiled, 1	0.6
Kidney, lamb, cooked, 100 g	0.4
Lamb, cooked, average serve, 150 g	0.2
Liver, cooked, 100 g	0.4
Pork, cooked, average serve, 150 g	0.2
Sausages, grilled, 2	0.4

Food	Vitamin E (milligrams)
Fish and seafood	
Eel, raw, 100 g	4.1
Fish, average fillet, grilled, 200 g	1.6
Fish, battered and fried, 1 piece, 160 g	1.9–16.0*
Fish, shallow fried in oil, 1 fillet, 150 g	3.5–10*
Herring, canned in tomato sauce, 100 g	3.6
Mussels, fresh, cooked, 10	1.1
Oysters, fresh, 6	0.8
Prawns, 100 g flesh, approx 4 large	2.9
Salmon, pink, canned, 100 g	1.5
Salmon, red, canned, 100 g	2.1
Salmon, grilled, 200 g	4.6
Sardines, canned in oil, drained, 100 g	0.3
Sardines, canned in tomato sauce, 100 g	3.1
Squid, in batter, 10 rings	2.3–4.0*
Tuna, canned in oil, 100 g	1.9
Tuna, canned in brine, 100 g	0.6
Tuna, fresh, 200 g	1.0
Nuts and seeds	
Almonds, toasted, 50 g	12.2
Brazil nuts, 50 g	3.6
Cashew nuts, plain or roasted, 50 g	0.7
Chestnuts, 50 g	0.6
Coconut, fresh, 50 g	0.4
Coconut, creamed, 50 g	0.7
Coconut milk	0
Hazelnuts, 50 g	12.5
Macadamia nuts, roasted, 50 g	0.7
Peanut butter, 1 tablespoon	1.0
Peanuts, 50 g	5.0
Peanuts, dry roasted, 50 g	0.6
Pecans, 50 g	2.2
Pine nuts, 50 g	6.8
Pistachio nuts, roasted, 50 g	2.2

* Quantity depends on type of fat or oil used

Food	Vitamin E (milligrams)
Poppy seeds, 2 teaspoons	0.3
Pumpkin seeds, 1 tablespoon	0.2
Sesame seeds, 2 teaspoons	0.2
Sunflower seeds, 1 tablespoon	7.6
Walnuts, 50 g	1.9
Fruit	
Apple, 1 average	1.0
Apricots, 2 average	0.7
Apricots, dried, 6	0.3
Avocado, $\frac{1}{2}$ medium	3.2
Banana, 1 average	0.3
Blackberries, $\frac{1}{2}$ punnet, 100 g	2.4
Blackcurrants, raw, 100 g	1.0
Cherries, 200 g	0.2
Fig, fresh, 1 medium, 60 g	0.5
Gooseberries, $\frac{1}{2}$ punnet, 100 g	0.4
Grapefruit, $\frac{1}{2}$ medium	0.3
Grapes, 200 g	trace
Kiwi fruit, 1 average	1.1
Loganberries, canned, $\frac{1}{2}$ cup	0.3
Mango, 1 average	1.5
Melon, 200 g slice	0.2
Olives, in brine, 10	0.9
Orange, 1 medium	0.4
Orange juice, 250 mL	0.4
Peach, 1 average	0.8
Pear, 1 medium	1.0
Pineapple, 1 slice, 150 g	0.2
Plums, 2 average	0.7
Prunes, 6	0.9
Raspberries, $\frac{1}{2}$ punnet, 100 g	0.5
Rhubarb, cooked, 1 cup	0.4
Strawberries, $\frac{1}{2}$ punnet, 125 g	0.3
Tamarillo, 1 medium	1.4

Food	Vitamin E (milligrams)
Vegetables	
Artichoke, globe, cooked, 100 g	0.2
Asparagus, steamed, 6 spears	1.0
Beans, broad, cooked, 100 g	0.4
Beans, green, cooked, 100 g	0.2
Broccoli, cooked, average serve, 100 g	1.1
Brussels sprouts, cooked, 6	1.0
Cabbage, green, cooked, 1 cup	0.3
Cabbage, green, raw, including outer leaves, 1 cup, 90 g	6.3
Cabbage, red, cooked, 1 cup	0.2
Capsicum, green or red, raw, 100 g	0.8
Carrot, mature, cooked, 1 medium	0.6
Cauliflower, cooked, 1 cup	0.1
Chinese greens, cooked, 1 cup	2.0
Eggplant, fried in oil, 100 g	5.5
Kale, cooked, 100 g	1.3
Leek, cooked, $\frac{1}{2}$ cup	0.6
Lettuce, 4 leaves	0.4
Mushrooms, fried in oil, 100 g	2.8
Mushrooms, raw, 100 g	0.1
Onion, baked, 1 medium	0.9
Onion, fried in oil, $\frac{1}{2}$ cup	1.3
Onion, raw, chopped, $\frac{1}{2}$ cup	0.4
Parsley, $\frac{1}{2}$ cup	0.5
Parsnip, cooked, 1 medium	1.6
Peas, green, cooked, $\frac{1}{2}$ cup	0.2
Peas, sugar snap or snow, 100 g	0.4
Potato, cooked, 1 average, 180 g	0.1
Potato, mashed, 1 cup	0.9
Potato chips, average serve, 200 g	2.0
Potato chips, oven-baked, 200 g	0.7
Pumpkin, average serve, 120 g	1.1
Pumpkin, butternut, average serve, 120 g	2.2

Food	Vitamin E (milligrams)
Spinach, English, raw or cooked, 100 g	1.7
Sweet corn kernels, canned, 1 cup	0.8
Sweet corn, cooked, 1 cob	0.8
Sweet potato, baked, 150 g	8.9
Sweet potato, cooked, 150 g	6.6
Tomato, raw, 1 medium, 150 g	1.8
Tomato juice, 1 cup	2.5
Tomato puree, $\frac{1}{2}$ cup	6.7
Watercress, raw, 1 cup	0.6
Legumes	
Beans, baked, 1 cup	0.7
Beans, haricot, cooked, 1 cup	0.1
Beans, kidney, canned, 1 cup	0.4
Chickpeas, cooked, 1 cup	2.2
Lentils, cooked, 1 cup	0.2
Soy beans, cooked, 1 cup	2.2
Split peas, cooked, 1 cup	0.6
Fats and oil	
Butter, 1 tablespoon	0.4
Canola oil, 1 tablespoon	4.4
Cod liver oil, 1 tablespoon	4.0
Corn oil, 1 tablespoon	3.4
Cottonseed oil, 1 tablespoon	8.6
Margarine, 1 tablespoon	0–5.6
Olive oil, 1 tablespoon	1.0
Palm oil, 1 tablespoon	6.6
Peanut oil, 1 tablespoon	3.0
Safflower oil, 1 tablespoon	8.1
Soy bean oil, 1 tablespoon	3.3
Sunflower oil, 1 tablespoon	9.8
Wheat-germ oil, 1 tablespoon	27.3
Miscellaneous	
Chocolate, 100 g	0.8

Food	Vitamin E (milligrams)
Mayonnaise, egg, homemade, 1 tablespoon	3.8
Popcorn, plain, oil popped, 1 cup, 10 g	1.1
Potato crisps, 50 g packet	1.6
Sausage roll, 1	1.8
Soy beverage, 1 cup	1.9
Tofu, 100 g	0.9

Effect of cooking

Considerable losses of vitamin E occur during storage and in cooking, and may amount to about 50 per cent of the initial levels. Freezing leads to some losses, and these vary with the food and the way it is packaged. However, most frozen foods are not significant sources of vitamin E, even when fresh.

Deficiency

In animals such as rats, a lack of vitamin E results in infertility. When this problem occurs in humans, it is not because of vitamin E deficiency. However, rhesus monkeys made experimentally deficient in vitamin E develop a degeneration of the nerves that control their muscles that is similar to one of the signs of a deficiency of vitamin E in humans.

Vitamin E deficiency does not occur in humans because of a dietary lack of the vitamin. However, it has occurred in the past in premature infants given a formula milk that was high in polyunsaturated fats (which increases the requirement for vitamin E) and high in iron (which acts as a pro-oxidant and increases the need for the antioxidant vitamin E). These infants, born with low tissue levels of tocopherol, suffered from the breakdown of their red blood cells (haemolytic anae-mia). Infant formulas for such babies now have higher levels of vitamin E. Some, but not all, of the many problems occurring in premature infants respond to vitamin E. An injection of vitamin E may prevent inter-cranial haemorrhage in very low birth weight infants. However, side effects of the large doses of vitamin E required are not known.

Vitamin E deficiency is more likely to occur when there is impaired absorption from the small intestine, as may occur with cystic fibrosis, short bowel syndrome, chronic cholestatic liver disease and with untreated coeliac disease. The worst cases occur when the flow of bile is impaired by severe disease. Even so, it takes several years before the level of vitamin E in adults is low enough to cause neurologic problems. The body stores five to ten years supply of vitamin E and this is probably a reason why deficiency is so rarely seen in adults. However, a deficiency due to liver disease in a young child will lead to symptoms in the developing nervous system. These include loss of deep tendon reflexes, poor balance and coordination, muscle weak-ness, impaired movement of the eyes, disturbances in the visual field and, possibly, cognitive development. Each of these symptoms can occur if there is damage from some other cause to sections of the spinal cord. If the problem is detected early, the symptoms are reversible.

Whenever fat absorption is impaired, there is a likelihood that vitamin E will also suffer. Some children with the rare disorder known as abetalipoproteinaemia fail to grow and have severe neurological problems, including impaired vision, because they cannot absorb fat. Some evidence shows that giving these children a low-fat diet plus extra vitamin E as a supplement can help.

There is great interest in what is often called a sub-clinical deficiency of vitamin E. Some claim that when blood plasma levels of vitamin E are on the low side of normal, people are more likely to develop clogged arteries and coronary heart disease, cancer, cataracts and various signs of ageing. Certainly, as discussed earlier in this chapter, there is some epidemiological evidence that people with lower levels of vitamin E in plasma have a higher incidence of atherosclerosis and certain types of cancer. However, until we have evidence from good clinical trials that vitamin E supplements can help prevent these conditions, they cannot really be said to be due to vitamin E deficiency.

In general, the plasma level of alpha tocopherol is used to give an indication of vitamin E status. Past advice was that a supplement should be used if plasma levels fall below 0.5 micrograms per millilitre. Many would now regard these levels are well below the threshold to define deficiency.

There is also some dispute as to whether the plasma level of alpha tocopherol is the best indicator of vitamin E status. The blood level tells you little about how well the vitamin is being transferred to and retained by the tissues.

With some people consuming high levels of polyunsaturated fats, and therefore needing much more vitamin E, there is a fear that deficiencies of this vitamin may become more common. In many cases, this fear is unlikely to be realised since many of the foods that are high in polyunsaturated fats are also high in vitamin E.

However, the increased need for vitamin E with high levels of polyunsaturated fats is yet another reason why it makes sense to keep these fats low, at least for those of the omega 6 series. Omega 3 polyunsaturated fats are found in fish and other seafood and also in linseeds. Products such as cod liver oil are also rich in vitamin E and most fish oil capsules have added vitamin E. However, some products from smaller vitamin manufacturers with poor quality control are potentially a risky choice. Linseed oil is also a potential risk. Although it is rich in vitamin E when pressed, the fatty acids in it are so unstable and oxidise so rapidly that the vitamin E may be used up by the high level of oxidative products that form within a short time after pressing. It makes more sense to eat linseeds than to use the oil. The seeds stick to the wall of the bowel for up to ten days while bacteria break them down and release their contents safely.

Excess

Vitamin E is not stored in the liver to any extent, but it is stored in body fat. It accumulates slowly and is released slowly if body fat breaks down to supply energy. Vitamin E is also stored in cell membranes and is carried in the body on lipoproteins (combinations of fat and protein). Most of the body's tocopherol is stored in muscle.

Unlike other fat-soluble vitamins, vitamin E is fairly non-toxic when taken by mouth. In theory, taking large doses of vitamin E could interfere with absorption of vitamins A and K. Taking more than 1200 milligrams of tocopherol a day (many hundreds of times the RDI) has been shown to interfere with the action of vitamin K in people taking anti-coagulants.

In general, there are no harmful effects from 200 to 800 milligrams of supplementary vitamin E, at least in the short term, although some people report gastrointestinal disturbances at the higher level.

Taking more than 800 to 1200 milligrams of vitamin E a day can lead to bleeding after surgery and it is not advisable to take high doses of vitamin E for several weeks before or after surgery.

There is danger in giving very small premature babies high doses of vitamin E intravenously or by injection. In the early 1980s, many premature babies died from a high-dose vitamin E preparation given intravenously, although this may have been due to the material that was used to keep the vitamin E in solution. This preparation is no longer available. High doses of vitamin E given orally to infants can cause a severe form of colitis.

Drugs

Many people take anti-coagulant drugs such as warfarin to thin the blood and prevent clots forming. There have been suggestions that taking vitamin E at the same time could change the effect of warfarin. However, one study giving up to 1200 IU a day (804 milligrams) found no effect on blood clotting time.

Vitamin E supplements

For vitamin E, this is a difficult question to answer. There is almost certainly a case for people with cystic fibrosis or any kind of malabsorption syndrome to use vitamin E supplements.

Whether those at risk of cardiovascular disease should use a vitamin E supplement is unclear. On the positive side, theoretical consideration of the way vitamin E may act and the advantages of preventing oxidation of fats, would suggest that a vitamin E supplement might be useful. On the negative side, the total confusion about an appropriate dose and the lack of proof from clinical trials means that a recommended safe and effective dose is unknown. With a couple of negative results, it would be wise to avoid taking huge doses, especially when there is no real proof that they are more effective than more modest quantities.

Once you start on vitamin E, there may also be a need for higher levels of vitamin C. This can easily be achieved from the diet. It may also make sense to ensure an adequate intake of vitamin E-rich foods as well.

In athletes

During strenuous exercise, tocopherol seems to be mobilised from the body's fat tissue and goes to the exercising muscles, presumably to prevent a build-up of oxidation products as the body burns fats as fuel. However, within a few minutes of stopping physical activity, tocopherol levels revert to normal. When vitamin E supplements have been given to athletes in controlled trials, no benefits have been shown. Activities involved in these trials have included bench-step tests, distance running, swimming, VO_2max, muscle strength, motor-fitness tests, cardiorespiratory efficiency during cycling tests. Under normal circumstances we can assume there is no benefit in athletes taking extra vitamin E.

However, testing athletes at altitudes of 1525 metres and 4570 metres, and giving them 1200 IU (800 milligrams) of vitamin E, showed that the supplemented group had lower levels of lactic acid in their blood and less oxygen debt. Researchers think that the lower availability of oxygen at altitude may cause greater breakdown of fats in the membranes around red blood cells. Acting as an effective antioxidant, extra vitamin E may counteract this.

Vitamin E supplements are often promoted to athletes on the basis that they will reduce muscle damage from strenuous exercise. Studies to test this theory have not given clear-cut results. Certainly, there is no reduction in muscle soreness in athletes taking 600 IU (400 milligrams) of vitamin E for several days before exercise. However, a couple of studies have shown less fat oxidation products in the blood of athletes who had taken 800 IU (536 milligrams) of vitamin E.

Current research findings

Research involving vitamin E is continuing on a large scale. An excellent summary of fairly recent research is published each year by Veris, a non-profit organisation. Funding for the publication of this work, however, does come from a large company involved in marketing the vitamin.

Research is currently concentrating on the following issues:

- how to determine vitamin E status in the body
- which forms of vitamin E supplements are best absorbed
- antioxidant activity and where it occurs in the body
- interactions with beta carotene and other carotenoids
- potential pro-oxidant activity of alpha tocopherol
- possible usefulness of vitamin E in preventing cataracts and other degenerative eye conditions
- vitamin E and the immune response
- usefulness of vitamin E for people with diabetes.

At this stage, the usefulness of vitamin E for these conditions needs confirmation from more studies before making claims.

6

Vitamin K

What it is

It's hard to think of alfalfa or decaying fish meal as desirable foods, but chickens who were deprived of these little tidbits bled so profusely that they developed fatal haemorrhagic disease. This situation occurred back in the 1930s, and in 1934 some Danish researchers found that alfalfa could cure the chickens' clotting problems. In 1939, one of the Danish researchers and a colleague from Switzerland isolated a fat-soluble substance which they called vitamin K (Koagulation vitamin).

Vitamin K exists in nature in two forms: phylloquinone, or vitamin K_1, in foods such as alfalfa and other green plants, and menaquinone, or vitamin K_2, which is made by bacteria. This was the form of vitamin K available from decaying fish, which is a rich source of bacteria. A third form of vitamin K, called menadione, is made synthetically and is often added to the feed of chickens and other animals to provide them with vitamin K.

The two natural forms of vitamin K are known by several names, and you may see these listed on supplements. The vitamin K from plants, K_1 or phylloquinone, is also called phytylmenaquinone and phytomenadione. When extracted from green plants, vitamin K_1 is a bright yellow oil which is soluble in fat.

In humans, vitamin K_2 is mostly made by bacteria living in the large intestine. Although it is difficult to study the production of vitamin K in the human intestine, most experts believe bacteria supply about half our vitamin K. The rest comes from the diet, and small quantities are found in some animal foods. Animals who eat their own faeces, such as rats, get their vitamin K from this source.

What it does

Vitamin K_1 is absorbed from the small intestine (from both the duodenum and jejunum) into the lymphatic system. It is then transported throughout the body. Anything that stops the absorption of fats can prevent vitamin K being absorbed.

We get about ten times as much vitamin K_2 from bacteria in the intestine as we get from foods, but the mechanism by which it is absorbed from the large intestine is not yet known. However, vitamin K_2 is found in the human liver, so we know that it is absorbed. Both types of vitamin K travel to the liver, with K_1 being used quickly and K_2 staying for longer. Any excess vitamin K is excreted in the faeces and urine. There is some evidence that vitamin K from foods is used more effectively than vitamin K from bacteria, but this is still largely unexplored.

It was not until the 1960s that researchers were able

to work out exactly what vitamin K does in the body. The vitamin is an essential cofactor in making four different proteins that are essential for normal clotting of blood. These are known as prothrombin or factor II, and factors VII, IX and X. Without vitamin K, if you cut yourself, you would bleed to death.

Much of the interest in vitamin K has come from infant health and nutrition. Before birth, an infant does not need vitamin K. At birth, very little vitamin K is transferred from the placenta and the newborn baby has very low levels of the vitamin. Its intestine also starts out sterile, so there is no synthesis of vitamin K by bacteria. Also, breast milk has low levels of vitamin K. It takes some time before the baby's liver will begin to make clotting factors. This means that if a newborn baby bleeds, the blood will not clot and the infant will have a massive haemorrhage. A spontaneous improvement takes place after the first week, but many maternity hospitals routinely give a newborn infant an injection of vitamin K as protection against any bleeding that may occur. However, even with the vitamin injection, the baby's liver may be slow to produce the clotting factor, prothrombin.

Some type of bleeding occurs in the first few days of life in one in every 800 infants. This may be either from trauma at birth, an injury to the skin, or from internal bleeding, usually somewhere in the gastrointestinal tract.

How much you need

In many countries, including Australia, no recommended dietary intake has been set for vitamin K. This is because there has been no way to determine how much of the vitamin is, or could be, made by bacteria in the intestine. In the United States, a Recommended Dietary Allowance has now been listed as 1 microgram of phylloquinone (vitamin K_1) per kilogram of body weight for adults. For infants, the recommendation is for 5 micrograms a day for the first six months of life and 10 micrograms a day after that. After one year of age, the same quantity as for adults (1 microgram per kilogram) is recommended.

Where it is found

The best sources of vitamin K are green vegetables such as broccoli, lettuce, cabbage, spinach and Asian greens. Amaranth leaves, used widely in parts of Asia, are especially high. Fats and oils contain small quantities. Meats, fish, dairy products and grains have very little. A few fruits are sources of vitamin K. Levels will be much higher in any fruits that are going 'off'.

Food	Vitamin K (micrograms)
Breads, grains and cereals	
Branflakes, 45 g	1
Bread, 2 slices	2
Cornflakes and other cereals, 45 g	negligible
Oats, raw, 50 g	2
Rice, white, raw, $\frac{1}{2}$ cup, 90 g	1
Rice cake, brown, 2	negligible
Spaghetti, uncooked, average serve, 100 g	negligible
Wheat flour, 1 cup, 125 g	1
Meat, poultry and fish	
Abalone, raw, 100 g	23
Beef	negligible
Fish, white flesh	negligible

Food	Vitamin K (micrograms)
Chicken	negligible
Egg, hen, 1 medium	1
Mackerel, 150 g	7
Pork	negligible
Salmon, 200 g	1
Yogurt, fruit, 200 g	1
Nuts and seeds	
Peanut butter, 1 tablespoon	3
Pistachio nuts, 50 g	35
Sesame seeds, dried, 2 teaspoons	1
Fruit	
Apple juice	negligible
Apple, with skin, green, 1 medium	6
Apple, without skin, raw, 1 medium	negligible
Apricots, canned, $\frac{1}{2}$ cup	6
Avocado, $\frac{1}{2}$ medium	40
Banana, 1 medium	1
Grapefruit, raw	negligible
Grapes, 200 g	6
Kiwi fruit, 1 medium	25
Melon, 200 g slice	2
Orange juice	negligible
Oranges	negligible
Peach, 1 medium	4
Plums, 2 medium	15
Vegetables	
Amaranth leaf, raw, 100 g	1140
Artichoke, raw, 1 average	21
Asparagus, raw, 6 spears	24
Beans, green, raw, 100 g	47
Beetroot, raw, grated, $\frac{1}{2}$ cup	2
Broccoli, cooked, 1 cup	270
Brussels sprouts, raw, 5 g	177

Food	Vitamin K (micrograms)
Brussels sprouts, top leaf only, 100 g	438
Cabbage, green, raw, 1 cup	130
Cabbage, red, raw, 1 cup	40
Capsicum, raw, $\frac{1}{2}$ medium	16
Carrot, cooked, 1 medium	16
Cauliflower, cooked, 1 cup	14
Cauliflower, raw, 100 g	5
Celery, raw, 2 pieces	5
Chives, raw, 1 tablespoon	10
Chinese greens, 1 cup	170–270
Coleslaw, $\frac{1}{2}$ cup	70
Coriander, fresh, $\frac{1}{2}$ cup	93
Cucumber, peeled, $\frac{1}{2}$ cup	1
Cucumber, with skin, $\frac{1}{2}$ cup	14
Endive, raw, 1 cup	126
Kale, raw, 1 cup	440
Kidney beans, dry, $\frac{1}{2}$ cup	18
Leek, raw, 1	17
Lentils, dry, $\frac{1}{2}$ cup	21
Lettuce, dark outer leaves, 2	210
Lettuce, inner leaves, 2	61
Mint, $\frac{1}{2}$ cup	75
Mushrooms, raw, 100 g	negligible
Nightshade leaf, cooked, 1 cup	1120
Onions, raw, 1 medium	3
Parsley, $\frac{1}{2}$ cup	173
Parsnips, 1 medium	1
Peas, green, cooked, $\frac{1}{2}$ cup	30
Peas, snow, 100 g	25
Pickles, dill, 1 pickle, 30 g	8
Potatoes, with skin, baked, 1 medium	7
Potato chips, average serve, 200 g	10
Pumpkin, mashed, $\frac{1}{2}$ cup	20
Pumpkin, with skin, average serve, 100 g	12
Pumpkin, without skin, average serve, 100 g	4

Food	Vitamin K (micrograms)
Purslane, raw, $\frac{1}{2}$ cup	152
Sauerkraut, canned, $\frac{1}{2}$ cup	30
Spinach leaves, raw, 1 cup	200
Spinach stalk, raw, $\frac{1}{2}$ cup	5
Spring onions, 2 average	120
Silverbeet, raw, 1 cup	450
Sweet corn, 1 cup	1
Tomato juice, canned, 1 cup	10
Tomato, ripe, raw, 1 medium, 150 g	9
Turnip greens, raw, 1 cup	150
Turnips	negligible
Watercress, raw, 1 cup	135
Fats and oils	
Almond oil, 1 tablespoon	1
Butter, 1 tablespoon	1
Canola oil, 1 tablespoon	28
Mayonnaise, 1 tablespoon	16
Olive oil, 1 tablespoon	10
Peanut oil, 1 tablespoon	negligible
Safflower oil, 1 tablespoon	2
Sesame oil, 1 tablespoon	1
Soybean oil, 1 tablespoon	39
Sunflower oil, 1 tablespoon	2
Walnut oil, 1 tablespoon	3
Miscellaneous	
Algae, purple laver, 50 g	690
Coffee, brewed, 1 cup, 150 mL	15
Potato chips, 50 g packet	5
Soy milk, 1 cup	8
Soybeans, dry, $\frac{1}{2}$ cup	45
Tea, brewed, 1 cup	negligible
Tea leaves, black, 2 teaspoons	10
Tea leaves, green, 2 teaspoons	60
Tofu, 100 g	2

Effect of cooking

Very little vitamin K is lost in cooking and cooked vegetables have as much vitamin K as raw ones. There is some loss of the vitamin in both acidic and alkaline solutions.

Deficiency

A deficiency of vitamin K is not common in humans, apart from the problems of haemorrhage in newborn babies. However, it does occur in conjunction with several other factors. As vitamin K is fat-soluble, any diseases that prevent absorption of fats can cause a deficiency. Use of antibiotics for more than a week is also a potential problem because the bacteria that make vitamin K are wiped out. If combined with a diet that has low levels of vitamin K, a deficiency can easily result. Anyone on long-term antibiotics who is not eating plenty of green vegetables should be monitored for low levels of vitamin K. Problems can also occur with people being fed through intravenous or naso-gastric tubes, if the mixture they are being given does not contain vitamin K.

Sometimes, vitamin K deficiency is also found in association with untreated coeliac disease, cystic fibrosis and short bowel syndrome. If the liver is severely diseased it may not make enough prothrombin, even if there is plenty of vitamin K available from the diet or from bacterial synthesis.

Drug interaction

Clover contains a substance called dicoumarol. If cattle eat too much spoiled sweet clover they can develop a tendency to bleed, because the dicoumarol stops the

normal production of clotting factors. Synthetic analogues of dicoumarol, such as warfarin, are used in
measured doses in humans to prevent blood clotting too
easily. Warfarin antagonises the action of vitamin K and
stops clotting factors being made in the body. For this
reason, when warfarin is being used to prevent blood
clots (or to 'thin' the blood), the dose is worked out
according to the person's current dietary intake of
vitamin K. This is why prescriptions of warfarin are
accompanied by an instruction leaflet telling you not to
make dramatic changes in intake of green vegetables.

Until recently, a deficiency of vitamin K was diagnosed by measuring the clotting time of blood, called
the 'prothrombin time'. This is a fairly insensitive measure of vitamin K status and more sensitive measure-
ments of clotting factors are being used. These allow a
mild deficiency of vitamin K to be diagnosed.

Excess

There do not seem to be any problems with high doses
of phylloquinone, the natural form of vitamin K. However, excessive doses of more than 1000 times the
requirement of the synthetic form of vitamin K, menadione, given to infants can cause haemolytic anaemia
and damage the liver.

Vitamin K supplements

Supplementary vitamin K is sold under the names
manphthone, phytomenadione, K-Thrombin and Konak-
ion.

Supplements of vitamin K, usually given by intramuscular injection, are important in preventing
haemorrhagic disease in newborn infants. Some of the

water-soluble forms of synthetic vitamin K can cause liver damage and are not suitable for infants.

Vitamin K is also given in severe liver damage or where there is some obstruction to the flow of bile.

People on large doses of anti-coagulants who experience bleeding (usually from gums or in stools) sometimes need vitamin K. The vitamin can be given by mouth or intramuscular injection.

Normal healthy people do not need supplements of vitamin K, although they are unlikely to be harmful.

Current research findings

Vitamin K acts as an essential factor to convert an amino acid called glutamic acid to another amino acid known as γ-carboxyglutamic acid. This acidic protein can then bind calcium and phospholipids which are necessary for the formation of thrombin. A protein containing residues of γ-carboxyglutamic acid, called osteocalcin, has also been isolated from bone. This protein and the blood clotting proteins that need vitamin K have many similarities. Researchers are now looking at their role in the movement of calcium into and out of bones. Vitamin D is also involved in these processes and the way the two vitamins may interact is being studied.

7

Non-vitamins and supplements

Over the years, many compounds have been described as vitamins. Some like vitamin H (now called biotin) have turned out to be vitamins. Many other compounds are still described as vitamins in books and health food literature, even though research has long since found they are not true vitamins. A few of these are described briefly here.

CAROTENOIDS

Beta carotene, already described in Chapter 1, is converted into vitamin A in the body. Some other members of the extensive family of carotenoid compounds can also be converted to vitamin A. Until recently, those carotenoids that were not converted to vitamin A were ignored. However, these abundant compounds that give colour to foods and flowers have other attributes which are unrelated to vitamin A. Medical researchers are now discovering their value.

Between 500 and 600 carotenoids have been identified (the variation in number is because some have very similar chemical configurations, and it is not always easy to tell if they are different, or simply different forms of the same compound). The major ones attracting attention at present are alpha carotene, beta carotene, lutein, zeaxanthin, cryptoxanthin and lycopene. These are discussed briefly in Chapter 1. As other carotenoids are studied, we can expect the list of valuable compounds to increase.

There are more than 200 studies showing that those who eat the most fruit and vegetables have the lowest levels of cancer at almost every site in the body. This protection does not come from the vitamins in these foods, or from the fibre. Researchers now believe the carotenoids (other than beta carotene) and other substances in plant foods may be responsible for the protection.

Carotenoids act as antioxidants, protecting the membranes around cells from damage inflicted by free radicals. Some may also stimulate the body's immune response. Other functions of specific carotenoids include normal functioning of detailed vision in the eye and an ability to prevent damaged cells from becoming malignant. Although they are important at all ages, most of these functions so far studied suggest they are even more important as people age.

A lot of evidence is already available about the usefulness of carotenoids. In one intervention study, 23 healthy men who did not smoke were given daily tomato juice (with 40 milligrams of lycopene), carrot juice (with

22.3 milligrams of beta carotene) and dried spinach with 11.3 milligrams of lutein. In all cases there was a decrease in damage to DNA in white blood cells. With the carrot juice, there was also a specific reduction in oxidative damage.

Blood samples from 7224 women in Missouri who had been blood donors over a ten-year period were analysed for levels of various carotenoids, as well as selenium, retinol and alpha tocopherol. Over the following years, 105 women diagnosed with breast cancer were found to have lower levels of lycopene, lutein, zeaxanthin and beta cryptoxanthin than a control group. There were no differences in levels of alpha or beta carotene, retinol, alpha tocopherol or selenium.

Heart attacks have also been shown to be inversely related to levels of lycopene in body fat in a major study from ten countries in Europe.

The most important aspect of the carotenoids may well be their diversity. It is highly likely that they exert their protective function when they act together. For this reason, taking pills containing one or two carotenoids is unlikely to have the same effect as eating a range of plant-based foods which will give you hundreds of them.

Some carotenoids, such as alpha carotene, may be destroyed by cooking. Others become more biologically available from cooked foods. The solution seems to be to eat a variety of plant foods, including both cooked and raw foods. This also makes good culinary sense, as some vegetables, in particular, are less palatable when raw.

There is no official recommended dietary intake for carotenoids. The many research studies being conducted into their benefits are intended to formulate supplements, so quantities that are safe and efficacious will no doubt be worked out in the near future. However, this is not necessary and may be counter-productive, if the experience with beta carotene is a guide. The best way to get enough carotenoids is to eat plenty of fruit and vegetables each day. Two to three pieces of fruit (the equivalent size of an orange) and at least five servings of vegetables ($\frac{1}{2}$ cup cooked or 1 cup raw) is a good start. More is even better. Try to include a wide variety of fruits and vegetables, and where possible, eat those that are in season. Tomatoes, for example, have their highest lycopene content when they are red and ripe.

B VITAMINS THAT AREN'T

Choline

Once thought to be a member of the B complex, choline lost this status as a vitamin when researchers found that humans could easily make it in their own bodies. Choline is an active constituent of lecithin, a compound made up of phosphorus and fat and found in foods as diverse as egg yolk and soybeans. Lecithin, and hence choline, is involved in the transport of fat within the body. Choline also plays a role in the way impulses are conducted along nerves and between nerves and muscles, although there is no evidence that taking choline supplements will help calm the nerves, as is sometimes claimed.

The idea that taking extra choline or lecithin will keep fats mobilised in the body and stop them being deposited in arteries or in fat stores on your hips or tummy are also false. Choline stops fats accumulating in the liver, but has no effect on fats being deposited anywhere else. Pills marketed as fat metabolisers often contain choline, but these products have no effect on deposition or loss of body fat. Lecithin can lower blood cholesterol, but only if given intravenously. Taken orally, as a supplement or as lecithin granules, it has no effect on blood cholesterol levels, probably because it is not absorbed from the intestine in this form. When lecithin granules appear to lower blood cholesterol, it is usually because the granules are made from soybeans and components in the soybeans (including the polyunsaturated fatty acids present) can lower undesirable cholesterol in the blood.

A lack of choline can occur, but is unlikely in anyone eating normal foods. If a deficiency does occur, it causes changes in liver cells and leads to fatty liver. Contrary to claims in some popular diet books, overweight people do not usually suffer from fatty liver, although it can occur in people whose livers have been damaged by certain strains of hepatitis or by excessive alcohol.

Good sources of choline in foods include liver, peanuts, vegetables such as cauliflower, lettuce, tomatoes and potatoes and wholegrain breads and cereals. Choline is also found in foods ranging from coffee to ice cream.

Carnitine

Once called vitamin B-T, carnitine is not a vitamin, but is made from two amino acids: lysine and methionine. It is found in foods and is also made in the body, where it is stored in skeletal muscle and in the heart.

Carnitine acts as a cofactor for an enzyme which transports long-chain fatty acids into the part of the cell where they can be oxidised as an energy source. As you might guess, some people have therefore assumed that taking extra carnitine as a supplement would increase the amount of fat burned for energy. Athletes and overweight people's hopes in this direction have been dashed by findings that extra carnitine from supplements cause the kidneys to reduce their efficiency in reabsorbing it.

Exercise does increase the amount of carnitine excreted, and some have suggested, therefore, that athletes need supplements. Several studies have reported a small benefit, but most have not. The form of carnitine in the body is L-carnitine. Supplements of D-carnitine can deplete the body's levels of L-carnitine and should not be taken. If you are tempted to take a supplement, and it does not state the type of carnitine present, resist the temptation.

Inositol

Once thought to be a member of the B complex, inositol turned out not to be a vitamin since it can be made by the body from glucose. It is part of a phospholipid (a combination of phosphorus and fat) and is part of the structure of cell membranes. High concentrations are found in the brain, heart and skeletal muscles, giving rise to the idea that athletes should take supplements. This idea has been put forward by Mark Colgan, who is often quoted in promotional material for inosine or inositol supplements. The 'study' quoted has not been published; it was conducted on four athletes and no statistical analysis of the supposed results was done. One valid study reported no benefits.

Orotic acid (vitamin B₁₃)

With full marks for its name (it is not a misprint), orotic

acid is important in RNA and DNA in the body and takes part in the synthesis of all body cells. In spite of such a useful role, orotic acid is not a vitamin because it is made in the body as needed. It is also found in milk, in the whey protein.

Pangamic acid (vitamin B_{15})

This substance, which is not a vitamin, was popular 20 to 30 years ago, when it was said to be responsible for the success of performances by Russian athletes. Various substances have been sold as pangamic acid, but the main one is a mixture of calcium gluconate (available in many calcium supplements) and dimethylglycine. One supplement was found to contain a substance called diisopropylamine dichloracetate which dilates the blood vessels, gives the body a 'kick' and causes blood pressure to drop. At least three studies using large doses of pangamic acid have been carried out with runners and with physically active men. None showed any value. If you come across pangamic acid, give it a wide berth.

Amygdalin (vitamin B_{17})

This substance was extracted from apricot kernels and promoted as a cancer cure at one stage. It is also marketed as laetrile and contains cyanide. It is likely that this may kill off some cancer cells, but unfortunately, it also kills the patient. Avoid it.

VITAMIN F

This substance is now known as alpha linolenic acid. Although it is essential in the body, it is not a vitamin but one of the essential omega 3 fatty acids. The richest source is linseeds (known as flaxseeds in some countries). Canola oil, walnuts and soybean oil contain small amounts. It is discussed further in the book *Good Fats, Bad Fats* (Rosemary Stanton, 1997, Allen & Unwin).

CHROMIUM PICOLINATE

Promoted as a supplement to increase muscle mass and reduce body fat, chromium picolinate is not a vitamin, but is often mistaken for one. Sellers of these supplements make many unsubstantiated claims, including the idea that it can increase lean muscle mass. There is no evidence to support this idea and studies making such claims were poorly controlled and conducted by someone who 'invented' chromium picolinate. Chromium is an essential mineral, but the value of chelating it to picolinate remains to be proven by independent investigators. So far, studies from these people have failed to replicate the benefits found by those who stand to make a profit from sales of the supplement.

FLAVONOLS

These are compounds belonging to the class of polyphenols and are found in the skin of grapes and some other fruits, and in red wine, tea and some vegetables. They function as antioxidants and seem particularly potent in preventing the oxidation of fats in the walls of the coronary arteries. However, purified flavonols do not have the same potency as those in products such as wine, so it may be that some of their action depends on other associated substances in the natural food sources.

FLAVANALS

A group of compounds belonging to the class of polyphenols which function as antioxidants. The most commonly consumed flavanals are the catechins found in green and black tea. Red wine also contains some, as do certain fruit skins and the barks of some trees.

Tea contains at least six different catechins, and the highest concentration is in young tea leaves. These compounds include catechin, epicatechin, gallocatechin, epigallocatechin, epicatechin gallate and epigallocatechin gallate. In making black tea, the green tea leaves are oxidised and some of the catechins form catechin quinones which then react to form theaflavins and thearubigens, compounds that give black tea its darker colour. Both these compounds are strong antioxidants, stronger than vitamins C and E. Flavanals and flavonols may have a role to play in protecting the body against oxidation reactions, but they should not be confused with vitamins.

SUPPLEMENTS

The wisdom or otherwise of taking vitamin supplements is discussed under each vitamin. The discussion here is intended to be more general.

There is little controversy about using vitamin supplements in cases of known deficiency. I certainly would not argue against adding extra vitamins to the diet of those in countries where malnutrition is common, although I would also like to see the ideal solution of greater food security addressed. But there is considerable debate about the wisdom and usefulness of adding supplementary vitamins to the diet of those who already have an adequate food supply.

Those who manufacture and market vitamins are, not surprisingly, in support of supplements. Some researchers are also supportive of additional vitamins, usually because of some epidemiological study results. The large Physicians Health Study in the United States, for example, found less coronary heart disease in men who had taken vitamin E tablets for many years compared with those who had not. Those who conducted this study therefore developed some enthusiasm for vitamin E supplements.

Such studies may show an association but do not offer proof. Real proof comes when studies look at two groups of evenly matched people, give one half the supplement in question and the other half a placebo pill, without either the researchers or the people themselves knowing which they are taking. The diets of both groups before and during the study also need to be accurately recorded. When the study code is broken, if the results between the two groups are dramatically different, and other factors have not been shown to change significantly between the groups, then and only then can you claim the supplement is effective.

The human race has survived well without supplements and life expectancy continues to increase, in spite of arguments that foods no longer provide nutrients or that the earth is so polluted that we need extra vitamins. Pollution is a great problem that we must address, but there is no evidence that taking large quantities of vitamins is needed to combat it.

Many studies have observed that those who eat the most fruit and vegetables have the lowest incidence of cancer at almost every site in the body. That does not mean, of course, that it is the vitamins in fruits and vegetables that are magic. It may be some of the other hundreds of compounds in fruits and vegetables—possibly even an extensive combination of these. Or it may be that people who eat fruits and vegetables also do other things that protect them from cancers. These studies have been discussed in Chapter 1.

Those promoting supplements often cite the results of large trials in the Linxian region of China where a combination of beta carotene, vitamin E and selenium led to a decrease in deaths from cancer of 13 per cent, a 9 per cent drop in strokes and 9 per cent fall in overall mortality. These were promising results but the population was deficient in these vitamins. Taking supplements to correct a known deficiency is quite different from taking them on top of an adequate diet where the supplement may well create an excess of the nutrient. With several large-scale randomised controlled trials using vitamin supplements showing adverse effects, it is important not to assume that if a little is good, more must be better.

Nutrition research is difficult to do and hard to interpret accurately. Results may be due to chance or to a faulty use of statistics. Even when a study is deemed to be statistically significant, there is still one chance in 20 that the results were due to luck. Many people gamble on far greater odds. Statistics can also be misused to imply a benefit that is not really there.

Also, there may be too many confounding factors. For example, if you find that vegetarians have less bowel cancer than meat eaters, is it because they get more vitamins from vegetables, or are there other factors in vegetables, or in nuts, soy products or fruits? Or is it something in the meat? It is also possible that vegetarians smoke less, drink less alcohol and coffee, take fewer painkillers or exercise more. Some of these factors may be totally irrelevant; others may be interrelated and it can be difficult to tease out any one factor.

Cause and effect can also be difficult to disentangle. Are people healthy because they take vitamins or are health conscious people more likely to take vitamins? And getting information about what people eat is fraught with error. People underestimate particular items, and questionnaires about how often you eat particular items are inaccurate because they miss so many items. Asking people to record what they eat also changes what they eat. Apart from the difficulty of collecting accurate information, it is difficult to translate it accurately.

In some vitamin studies, the dose or combination given may also be wrong. For example, giving too much of some antioxidant nutrients can cause them to act as pro-oxidants.

All in all, research to show benefits from supplements does not always live up to what is expected of scientific research. The conclusion must be that humans do better eating a variety of healthy foods—as has been discussed for each of the true vitamins.

Index